362.1

Creating Moments of Joy

November 2003

Creating Moments of Joy
for the Person with
Alzheimer's or Dementia

A Journal for Caregivers

by Jolene Brackey

Purdue University Press / West Lafayette, Indiana

04   03   02   5   4   3

♾ The paper used in this book meets the minimum requirements of American National Standards for Information Sciences—Permanence of Paper for Printed Library Materials, ANSI Z39 48-1992.

Printed in the United States of America.

Library of Congress Cataloging-in-Publication Data available.

To my mom and dad—

for your love,
faithfulness and
for giving me
wings to fly.

Contents

How to Use This Journal	xi
Acknowledgments	xv
Prelude	1
Understanding the Person with Alzheimer's	3
Powerful Tools that Create Positive Outcomes	
Living Their Truth	9
Universal Reasons	13
"I want to go home"	17
Sense of Belonging	20
"Help me "	23
Magic Words	27
You Are Wrong, They Are Right	29
Blame It on Something or Someone Else	33
Let's Talk Communication	
Let's Talk Communication	39
Find the Treasures	44
Quality Connections	47
Take Action!	51
The Illusion of Choice	55
Your Mood Affects Their Mood	58
Look Good, Feel Good, Play Good	61
The Power of Touch	65
Kick Starting	68
Memory-Enhanced Environments	
Trigger Fond Memories	75

Create a Safe Haven   79
Life Reflection   82
Replacing Priceless Treasures   85
Fill Habits of a Lifetime   88
Music Does Wonders   91
A Commercial about TV   95
Where's the Outhouse?   98
It's Saturday Night! Bath Time!   101

Enhanced Moments
Simple Pleasures   111
You've Got Mail!   114
Walking, Walking, Walking   117
When In Doubt . . . Laugh   122
Share Your Life   125
Drink Up!   129
Saturating Obsessions   131
Spread Holidays throughout the Year   134
Keys to Visiting   139
Saying Good-Bye   143
Outings with Less Stress   146
Face the Challenges   150
Letting Go of Expectations   160
Spiritual Well-Being   164
Find the Blessings   169
Taking Care of Yourself   173

Conclusion   179

Bibliography   183

Index   185

Meet the Author   187

This journal belongs to

_____

who lives at

_____

_____

_____

I, _____ ,

am the primary care person and I live at

_____

_____

_____

my phone number is: (_____)_____.

If you want to know more about us, just look inside this book, and you will open the window to our hearts.

Create a Moment of Joy!

How to Use This Journal

I have a vision, a vision that we will soon look beyond the challenges of Alzheimer's disease and focus more of our energy on *creating moments of joy*. When a person has short-term memory loss, his life is made up of moments. But if you think about it, our memory is made up of moments, too. Think back to one of your fondest memories—family vacation, childhood friend, favorite pet. What do you remember, the day or the moment? It's the moment we remember. When you create a moment of joy for someone else, you are creating a memory for yourself.

This book offers many ways to create moments of joy. No matter what your environment or situation is, this book will be a positive tool on a daily basis.

I have broken down the learning process into five sections. Within those sections are smaller steps. At the end of each step is a place where you can journal your thoughts, solutions, and treasures. With this journal, you will gradually achieve the overall goal of creating many moments of joy.

Understand the Person with Alzheimer's — This is your foundation. You need to understand where the person believes she is living in her mind before you can respond appropriately.

Powerful Tools That Create Positive Outcomes — Here's where you begin to understand how a person with dementia communicates with you. This section includes tools you can use to offer comfort when he approaches you with his daily struggles. These tools will enable you to react to his questions and statements.

Let's Talk Communication — Now you can learn how to initiate effective communication by using a proactive approach. Once you find the treasures that each individual holds, you will enhance her life by reminding her who she is and also by knowing what makes her feel good.

Memory-Enhanced Environments — In this section you will discover what triggers a sense of comfort for the person with Alzheimer's. When he is comfortable, he will find peace in their environment.

Enhanced Moments — Discover the daily activities that will bring back joy to the person and to you!

If I can have you take just one thing with you after reading this book, I hope it is the courage to try everything once. You will make mistakes. Mistakes are valuable because they are stepping stones for all your successes. As long as you keep trying, there is still hope—hope to find the treasures that work. Discover the different tools that will help you dig for these treasures. When you find the treasure, write it down at the end of each step. Now practice, practice, practice.

Once you create a new habit for yourself, move onto another step. Let go of all your expectations and savor the simple surprises you receive along the way. When the time comes, pass this journal along, filled with your solutions and treasures. I bet the treasures you discover will create moments of joy for other people as well. Scribble notes anywhere and everywhere about anything at all, so your loved one's wants and wishes are not lost but bound together in this personal journal.

It is also my true desire to create moments of joy for you, the person who holds and reads this book. I have carefully selected stories, quotes, and dashes of humor in the hope that you will remember, cry, laugh, and love. When you see a twinkle in your loved one's eyes or comfort on her face, consider this your pat on the back. You did it! You created a moment of joy!

> *When we learn with pleasure, we never forget.*
> — Alfred Mercier

I'd love to hear from readers who have had success creating special moments of joy, so that we could include them in future editions of this book. Your sharing will really help others to help their loved ones. Please contact me at the address on the last page of this book.

Acknowledgments

To the people with Alzheimer's disease — for touching my life daily.

To the CNAs and activity directors — for passing on all your wonderful ideas. You have "It."

To Deb and Kate — for being my guiding lights.

To my close friends — for believing in me and giving me fond memories filled with joy.

To Jeanne — for your shared passion, valuable input in this book, and for your vision for the future.

To Ron Kitterman — for your understanding of spiritual well-being. It is the glue that holds my words together.

To Lori — for your words of wisdom and encouragement.

To Julie Granger and Paula Davis — for not only editing my book but feeling my emotions.

To Heidi — for patiently offering insights on how to wrap up my thoughts.

To Terry — for capturing my thoughts into drawings.

To David — for the opportunity to fulfill my dreams.

To Teresa — for sharing this adventure with me.

To my family — together we are a foundation solid as a rock.

To Troy, Sidney and Taylor — You are my treasures!

I would like to gratefully acknowledge all of the writers whom I have quoted for their wisdom and inspirational words. If there is an error concerning permission to reprint, I apologize, and a correction will be made in subsequent editions.

Creating Moments of Joy

Prelude

Bob was an avid fly fisherman and loved fishing the streams of Oregon. I met Bob when he moved into our facility after being diagnosed with Alzheimer's. He had a wonderful relationship with his wife. I asked her to bring me one of Bob's fishing poles. We were all outside enjoying the sun when his wife opened the door with a fishing pole in her hand. I gave the pole to Bob and asked if he would show us how to cast. He tossed the line out with such ease and then handed me the fishing pole. Needless to say, I didn't do very well, but he enjoyed watching me try. Then I asked him, "How do you tie the lures on?" He grabbed into the air for a fishing line, which wasn't really there, and he moved his hands and fingers as if he were tying the knot. He looked over at me with the imaginary knot in his hand and a smile on his face. I said, "You're amazing," and he just laughed.

This is what I mean by "creating a moment of joy." Bob relived one of his own simple pleasures, fly fishing—a pastime he loved. If his wife hadn't brought in his fishing pole, this moment would not have occurred. We would have missed our opportunity to create a moment of joy. Instead we captured it. We created a moment of joy for the residents who were watching, a moment of joy for me, for his wife, and, most importantly, a moment of joy for him.

Understanding
the Person with Alzheimer's

A person with Alzheimer's will lose short-term memory but retain long-term memory if we learn how to trigger it. The first part of the brain that is damaged affects the short-term memory. This is why he repeats his stories, why he cannot remember what he had for breakfast or that his son visited last night. When you ask him what he had for breakfast, he says, "I didn't have breakfast. Would you make me some?" Switch to his long-term memory and ask what he likes to eat for breakfast, cereal or eggs?

Another classic situation is when you say something like, "I heard your son came to visit you last night." The response goes like this, "What! Where was he? He didn't come see me." Again, switch to her long-term memory and tell her how you met her son, Eric, the other day and that she must be a wonderful mother because he is such a gentleman.

During a discussion about pets, Tom piped up about his pet mule. He said, "I had a pet mule once named Topsie. The only way to get Topsie to work for me was to share my tobacco with him." I asked him how old he was, and he said, "I was about fifteen or sixteen." Tom is eighty-two years old and doesn't remember what he had for breakfast, but he still remembers details from his childhood. He not only remembered how old he was and the name of his

mule, but he remembered how to get Topsie to work
for him. That's a treasure!

People who are in the early stages of Alzheimer's cannot remember how to make coffee or have difficulty finding
their way home. But when they visit the place where they
grew up, they comment how memories trickle out as if it
were yesterday.

As the Disease Progresses, Age Regresses

As the disease progresses, persons with Alzheimer's get
younger and younger and younger in their mind. In other
words, early in the disease they may have only lost the last
twenty years, but as the disease progresses they may lose
the last forty years, the last sixty years, and so on. This is
why they don't recognize their spouse—in their mind they
think they are twenty-five and their spouse is too old to be
their spouse. They may ask where their mom is or get up
and want to go to school.

If they begin talking in the mirror, they think they are
really talking to another person because they don't recognize themselves. That person in the mirror is much older
than they are. Talking to a mirror may have a negative effect
because the person in the mirror doesn't talk back or may
look ill; such a situation needs to be monitored. People with
Alzheimer's even revert back to their native language. If
they lived in Germany until they were fifteen years of age,
they might start speaking German again. If you no longer
understand what they are saying, rule out whether or not
they are talking in their native tongue. If they are talking in
German, it may be beneficial to learn to say everyday
words in German.

How do you figure out what age they are living? The
simplest way is to ask them, "How old are you?" If they do
not respond or show confusion answering this question,
there are other ways to figure out what age they believe
they are living. If they are looking for their spouse but do
not recognize him or her, you can assume they remember

they are married—which is usually between the age of twenty to forty. If they are constantly talking about or looking for their mom, you can assume they are an adolescent. If they are looking for their children and do not recognize their children, you can assume they are in younger adulthood—perhaps early twenties or thirties. Once you figure out what age they are living, then figure out what was significant in their life at that time and use that information to create moments of joy.

> *I heard a story about a gentleman who angrily walked around yelling, "horse! horse!" The staff labeled him as agitated and usually avoided him because his yelling was so annoying. They eventually decided to talk to the family about this "behavior." The family replied that when he was in his twenties he took care of horses. With this understanding, they brought in a saddle, reins, appropriate cleaning supplies, and pictures of horses and filled his room with items familiar to him. His yelling diminished, and he would clean the saddle and reins for long periods of time.*

It's exciting! Once we understand why a person with dementia does what he does, then we accept the challenges with a positive outlook. We now have energy to find a solution instead of dwelling on the problem. "Behaviors," or more positively called "actions and reactions," are windows to a person's mind, and we can help bring light to that window.

Change with the Pearl

"Our value lies in what we are and what we have been, not in our ability to recite the recent past."

—Homer, a man with Alzheimer's disease

New-Found Understanding

_____

_____

_____

_____

_____

_____

_____

_____

_____

_____

_____

_____

_____

_____

_____

_____

_____

_____

_____

_____

_____

_____

_____

_____

_____

_____

_____

Powerful Tools
That Create
Positive Outcomes

Love and care with a genuine heart.

Living Their Truth

Since a person with Alzheimer's has lost the last twenty to sixty years, she may be living around the 1940s in her mind. No matter how hard we try, we cannot bring back her short-term memory. We can, however, take hold of her long-term memory and use it to create moments of joy. This means we need to live her reality. When she is looking for her mom, we need to tell her that her mom is at church or getting groceries. By giving answers that make sense to her, she is able to relax and not worry about where her mom is.

You might not like doing this because you think you are lying to them. I assure you it is not lying; it is "living their truth." When you live their truth, your body language and tone of voice need to be genuine and "matter of fact," so the person believes what you are saying. If you hesitate or look confused, the person with dementia will sense this and may become suspicious.

Maybe it will help if you visualize yourself in her position. You have Alzheimer's but do not remember you do, and you think you are perfectly fine. You are actually eighty-five but think you are twenty-four. You wake up every morning in a strange place. You remember you have children, but you cannot find them. You ask a stranger who acts as if they know who you are, "Where are my children?" She tells you the truth: "Your daughter isn't visiting until Tuesday. You live here now. Everything will be fine." Your reaction would be: "Everything will not be fine because this is not my home, and I think you are lying to me. I want to go home! I need to find my children." Does this vision help you understand? More importantly, I hope it takes away some of the guilt you feel about "lying." The bottom line is this: there is no reasoning with a person who has Alzheimer's, and you will not be able to make her live your reality. You can fight until you are blue in the face, but one way or another she will win in the end. Live her reality and find treasures in her reality. Once you start doing this, the person with Alzheimer's will take you on some wonderful cheap adventures. While on these adventures, collect treasures from her long-term memory and give the treasures back every day after that. When you "live their truth," I guarantee more positive, productive days lie ahead of you.

> *Margaret would wake up in the morning and want to water her horse. I would whisper (because it's our little secret), "I got up early and did it for you. You can sleep in this morning." Now, we all know what happens to kids when they don't do their chores. If I had told Margaret she no longer has a horse, she would worry about what had happened to it.*

> *Jack would wake up at 4:00 A.M. almost every morning and insist he had to go to work. He was a construction worker most of his life, and until people "lived his truth," he would become combative because staff members insisted he did not have to work anymore. They needed to give him a universal reason why he did not have to go to work. Now the answer is, "It's raining out. Your crew called and said it's too wet to work. If you would like, I will make you some coffee or you can go back to bed." Notice we didn't make him go back to bed, because his "habit of a lifetime" was getting up at 4:00.*

I hear and I forget. I see and I remember.
I do and I understand.
— Chinese Proverb

New-Found Truth and How You Lived It

_____

_____

_____

_____

_____

_____

_____

_____

_____

_____

_____

_____

_____

_____

_____

_____

_____

_____

_____

_____

_____

_____

Universal Reasons

Whatever age the person with Alzheimer's is living, we need to give him a reason why he doesn't have to do what he thinks he has to do. Give him a universal reason "why" or at least something that he may believe. The following are statements/questions that are asked repeatedly. Of course, you need to apply each answer on an individual basis.

Where are my children?

If the person thinks she has young children who are still dependent on her, you need tell her a story to let her know her children are OK.

Possible Answers:

Your kids are in school.

Your kids are at ——'s house.

Your kids are taking a nap upstairs. They just fell asleep.

I have to go to work.

Possible Answers:

It's a holiday.

It's Saturday.

The boss called and said he wouldn't be in, so you are to take the day off.

I need to go to school.
 Possible Answers:
   It's suppose to storm today so they cancelled
   school.
   It's a holiday.

Where is my mom?
 Possible Answers:
   She is running errands.
   She is getting groceries.
   She is shopping.
   She is over at ——'s house.

Where is my husband?
 Possible Answers:
   He is at work.
   He is uptown with ——.
   He is out in the field.
   He is at the hardware store.

Where is my wife?
 Possible Answers:
   She is at church.
   She is getting her hair done.
   She is visiting ——.
   She is getting groceries.

Another very difficult situation is when the person asks where his spouse is, and his spouse has already passed away. Again, we need to live his reality. First realize that the person would not be asking where his spouse is if he didn't think she was alive. When we tell him his wife is no longer living, it would be like someone telling you today that your spouse is no longer living. You would deny it because you just saw him this morning. You would be angry because no one told you that he died. You would have grief and depression. Now imagine that you asked that question every day. It would definitely affect your health and decrease functioning ability. I cannot stress enough that you should not tell the person that his spouse has passed away. Instead think of what his spouse might be doing if she were alive. "Alice is getting her hair done." "Beth is at work." "Joe is out in the field plowing." Anytime you can fill in the names of people and what they would actually be doing during the day, your story is obviously more believable. If you don't know the answer to the question, then ask him, "What does your wife do during the day?" Then the next time he asks, you have a believable answer. If there is more than one care provider, make sure you all have the same story. Jot it down for all staff to see and train new staff on these answers. When the person with dementia gets different answers (stories) to his questions, he might become more confused, and your story isn't worth much.

Be like a duck . . . keep calm and unruffled on the surface
but paddle like the devil underneath.

—Unknown

New-Found Universal Reason

_____

_____

_____

_____

_____

_____

_____

_____

_____

_____

_____

_____

"I want to go home."

The guilt that families feel when they hear "I want to go home" sometimes compels them to move a loved one into their home, thinking it will help. Families may also stop visiting because it becomes too uncomfortable. However, the "home" that the person with dementia is looking for no longer exists because it is a home from long ago. Even if you took him home, he will still want to go home. Saying "I want to go home" could also mean he is looking for the feeling of home: love, laughter, security, and sense of belonging. The best thing we can do is to help the person with dementia to feel safe and comfortable in the place he needs to live in.

Possible Answers

Distraction — *"Tell me about your home. Do you live on a farm or in town?"*

Support — *"Your brother will pick you up at ——."*

Magic words — *"I know things are a bit confusing right now, but I will be here if you need me. I care about you, ——."* (It helps if you use body language to assure the person by putting your hand over her hand and giving it a gentle squeeze.)

Reason — *"The doctor wants to make sure you are feeling 100% better, so he thought you should stay one more day."*

(In earlier generations the doctor was put on a pedestal and was not usually questioned.)

For a person with dementia, typically around 3:00 P.M. it's time to go home because in her truth she needs to be home for dinner. You need to give her a reason to stay. For instance, you can say, "Stay for supper, I made a special meal for you." Then after supper, your answer may be, "It's late, please just stay the night. I have a room all ready for you." If she needs more reassurance or is worried others will wonder where she is, you can add, "I called your daughter/mom and she said she would pick you up in the morning."

Be aware of the telephone ringing in the background. It may trigger the person with Alzheimer's to want to call someone or want to go home. Having a phone in her room triggers her to call family many times a day. The family member now becomes the victim. Reduce the number of calls to family by creating a busy signal or constant ring on the other end to convey no one is home. Give her a reason "why" there isn't a phone in her environment. "The phone is getting fixed." Be there for families!

It seems to me that our basic needs,
for food and security and love,
are so entwined
that we cannot think of one without the other.
—M. F. K. Fisher

New-Found Response to "I Want to Go Home"

_____

_____

_____

_____

_____

Sense of Belonging

Any human being would feel some level of fear and insecurity if she were in an unfamiliar place with people who did not seem to have answers to her questions. We need to provide answers that will make the person feel like she belongs "here." For some, this will never really be "home," and you should realize that they won't ever want to stay "here," but it might be OK to stay a little longer. If they feel this arrangement is temporary, they are more likely to relax and enjoy their day. For some people the blessing is they think they have lived "here" for two weeks, but actually it has been two years.

> *"Where are my children?" Now, we knew Sarah had a strong work ethic, so the answer that usually worked was: "Ted is working downtown, and Shirley will pick you up at 5:00 P.M." Ted actually did work downtown, and if Sarah had a good morning she would be OK with Shirley picking her up at 5:00. If she wasn't having a good day, she would usually respond, "I raised and took care of those kids; they better take care of me. I am not staying here until 5:00." Because of her short-term memory loss, she would come around the corner within thirty seconds and ask the same question to the same person. If she was upset, we knew we needed to change our response: "Ted is at work, and Shirley just called and said she*

is picking you up at 10:00 this morning." Then at 10:00 we would say Shirley was picking her up at 12:00; at 12:00 she was picking her up at 4:00; at 4:00 she was picking her up after supper; after supper she was picking her up at 8:00; at 8:00 she was picking her up in the morning. You knew that Shirley wasn't really going to pick her up. Shirley is really coming on Tuesday to take her out for lunch, but if we told her that, she would get extremely upset. This will never be her home and she will always want her kids. This answer helped her enjoy her time with us.

This technique should not be used for people who still have short-term memory. For example, if you tell a person who has short-term memory that someone will be coming at noon to pick her up, but someone really isn't coming until Tuesday, she will be sitting by the door, waiting all day. Different dementias affect people in a variety of ways.

> *Kind words can be short and easy to speak,*
> *but their echoes are endless!*
> — Mother Teresa

New-Found Sense of Belonging

_____

_____

_____

_____

_____

_____

_____

_____

"Help me"

Whatever your task may be, ask the person with dementia to help you. Human beings have an innate desire to feel needed—and more so with older generations, who were brought up to help one another. Encouraging the person with dementia to be responsible for the home might make it seem more like "home."

> I asked two ladies to help me set the table. They lined up the glasses on one table, stacked place mats here and there, plates were randomly placed on the tables and one of the ladies started folding and rubbing the napkins. I could have corrected them and said, "That's not where the glasses go. Glasses go above the plates." But instead I said, "Oh thanks so much for all your help. Why not relax in the living room while I finish dinner? I'll call you when it's ready." After they left, I easily set the tables the right way. Not only did they "help" me, but they were a part of the meal preparation, which triggers the experience that it will soon be time to eat. If you are concerned about sanitation, purchase at a thrift store an extra set of dishes just for the residents, so they can help rinse and wash dishes too.

Have your loved one help you clean a closet, cut out coupons, move boxes, make beds, sweep the patio, rake leaves, hang clothes, wipe furniture, wash dishes, fold laundry, peel oranges, sort cards, roll yarn, stack wood, shell corn to feed the squirrels, water the garden, snap beans, de-stem strawberries, polish and sort silverware, crack peanuts, tear lettuce for a salad, butter bread—the list goes on forever. Create things for her to do even if it doesn't need to be done. The key is to choose something she has done frequently in the past. And guess what . . . you can offer the same projects every day, because she doesn't remember she did it the day before. One of my favorites was rolling up yarn. Once a week, I would pull out a box of yarn, unroll it and bring it into the living room and say, "I found this in the closet, and it's a mess. Would you help me roll this yarn up?" Men helped, too, because they like to help the ladies.

Simplify, simplify, simplify every task to ensure less stress and more success. Let go of any expectations. A good example of this is if you asked your loved one to help you weed the garden, and she pulls up a few flowers. Stop and think, "Who cares?" The flowers cost only pennies. The important part is to trigger her experience of gardening, something she may have always enjoyed doing. Let go of having to do things the way they have always been done. Not only are you providing exercise, relieving stress, and making the person feel useful, but also you are creating a moment of joy.

Asking for her advice is another way to reinforce the feeling she is still needed. Don't expect a logical clear answer. You are giving a greater gift by fulfilling the desire to be needed, wanted. No expectations attached!

I learned early on that setting a table is so much more than just laying down knives and forks. It is creating a setting for food and conversation, setting a mood and an aura that lingers long after what was served and who said what was forgotten.

—Peri Wolfman

New-Found Job Your Loved One Likes to Help With

_____

_____

_____

_____

_____

_____

_____

_____

_____

_____

_____

_____

_____

_____

_____

_____

_____

_____

_____

_____

_____

_____

_____

Magic Words

When you are really upset about something, isn't it wonderful to have a friend to call who knows just what to say to make you feel better? We feel better when people around us are supportive, caring, and thoughtful. Our troubles seem to lessen when we have others to lean on. When a person with dementia is troubled, try to think of magic words to make him feel better if you were in his shoes.

Examples of Magic Words

I will be here all day if you need anything.

Don't worry, I'll take care of it.

You are pretty important around here.

If you need anything, just let me know.

I do silly things like that too.

Between the two of us, we will be OK.

You are a pretty special person.

Modern science is trying to produce a tranquilizer more effective than a few kind words.

—Unknown

New-Found Magic Words

_____

_____

_____

_____

_____

_____

_____

_____

_____

_____

_____

_____

_____

_____

_____

_____

_____

_____

_____

_____

_____

_____

_____

_____

You Are Wrong, They Are Right

Stop correcting people with dementia! This may be hard to swallow, but they are always right, and you are always wrong. When you are always wrong and they are always right, there is nothing to fight about. You will usually end up with quicker resolution instead of confrontations. Once you accept this, you are essentially on a new road to build up their self-esteem. We absolutely need to stop correcting them. It only reminds them that they are not OK. We think by correcting them we are setting them on the "normal" path again, but the best thing we can do is reassure them that they are OK right now. When everyone around them is supportive and agrees with them, they start to feel OK. In return, this will build their confidence, their self-esteem, and their independence.

Ways We Constantly Correct Our Loved Ones

No, Mom, you live here now and Dad has passed away.

I told you ten times you had a doctor appointment.

Helen, I am your husband. Don't you remember me?

Bob, this is not your room.

No, Dad, I am your son, John.

29

Mary, those aren't your clothes.

Don't you remember?

You already told me that story.

You are retired and don't have to work anymore.

Ways to Make Them Feel OK

• **Being in someone else's room:** When we see a person with Alzheimer's rummaging in someone else's room, our natural reaction is to say, "Alice, this is not your room. You need to come out, and I will take you to your room." Do you think she would be in that room if she knew it wasn't her room? Absolutely not! Do not correct her, but give her a reason to leave the room: "Alice, would you help me in the kitchen for a minute?" "Joe, could you help me move some boxes?" Obviously, choose a task the person enjoys doing.

• **Wearing layers of clothing or someone else's clothing:** It is very hard for a person to get dressed once, let alone twice. Instead of trying to change his clothes, let him wear the clothes for the day and return them to the rightful owner after he gets ready for bed. Ask yourself this: Would he have ever worn someone else's clothes before dementia? A positive aspect of Alzheimer's facilities is that the other residents usually do not know someone else is wearing their clothes. If you have no other choice but to take off a piece of clothing, give him a logical reason why. For example, "Joe, I found this other sweater. Not only is it warmer but it will really look good on you," or "Boy, it's hot in here. I bet you would feel better if you took off your sweater."

- **Repeating stories:** Patience, patience, patience. Patience is a virtue but difficult to have twenty-four hours a day. Get the person involved in something she enjoys doing: peeling potatoes, snapping beans, folding clothes, cracking nuts, shucking peanuts, sorting through a tackle box, etc. Maybe there is something in her environment that triggers a certain story, so you may want to remove it. Another hint is to find a short, simple response: "That's interesting." Repeat the response that works. (If you need to take a break, give a universal reason why you need to leave the room. My all-time favorite is, "I need to go to the bathroom. I will be right back." Even if you do not have to use the bathroom, you need time out.) Try not to respond with, "You already told me that story." She does not remember, and you are only reminding her that something is wrong.

Imagine, if you will, going into a grocery store and strangers coming up to you. They tell you you're wearing someone else's clothes, that you can't go down that aisle, or that you are picking out the wrong food. People are constantly correcting you and telling you no. Would you want to stay in the grocery store? No, you would probably want to go home. This is how a person with dementia feels when we constantly correct her. Understand that she is doing the best she can with the abilities she has left. We are the ones who have to change, because they are unable to.

When they are doing something that isn't normal, here is one way to decide whether or not to correct them. Ask yourself these three questions. Is it hurting them? Is it hurting you? Is it hurting anyone at all? If the answer is no to all of these questions, then you let them do what they want to do.

Their biggest stress is us asking them to be normal.
We are going to have to change because they are unable to.
—Moyra Jones

New-Found Right Made Wrong

_____

_____

_____

_____

_____

_____

_____

_____

_____

_____

_____

_____

_____

_____

_____

_____

_____

_____

_____

_____

_____

_____

_____

_____

_____

_____

Blame It on Something
or Someone Else

Another wonderful way to make everyone happy is to blame mistakes on something or someone else—administrators, spouses, the environment. Blame it on yourself by saying, "I'm sorry. It's my fault," or "Oh yeah, you're right. I forgot." Your greatest gift is to make the person feel OK because all he really needs is someone who understands and accepts him as he is!

- **Forgetting appointments:** You know that people with dementia have short-term memory loss, and to compensate you call your loved one ten times in the morning to remind her of a doctor's appointment, and you also leave a written note on the refrigerator. When you arrive to pick her up, you begin saying, "Are you ready to go to the doctor?" The answer is, "You didn't tell me I had a doctor's appointment. I am not ready to go anywhere." Then, being only human, we tend to lose our patience altogether and say, "I told you ten times and left you a message. Your appointment is today." This statement is an instant reaction expressing your frustration, but you are only making her upset, confused, and reluctant to go with you. A much better response is to blame yourself for this misunderstanding. It's

33

hard to be wrong, but just do it: "Oh no, I forgot to tell you. I thought I did. I'm sorry. But can we still make the appointment?" Would you like another little hint? Don't take the time to remind her, but just apologize for "forgetting" when you pick her up, and arrive early, knowing she may need help getting ready.

• **Incontinence:** It can be very embarrassing for a person with dementia to wake up in the morning and find the bed is wet. Blame it on something else. "That roof is leaking again! I can't believe it! I have to get it fixed." This answer really works! Now he thinks he didn't wet the bed or he thinks he has you "snow balled." If the person is incontinent during the day, blame it on something else. "You must have sat in some water. Let's change those pants so you'll feel better."

Patient: Doc, I broke my finger in two places.
Doctor: Well, stay out of those two places.

New-Found Thing to Blame It On

_____

_____

_____

_____

_____

_____

_____

_____

_____

Let's Talk Communication

Take things lightly and you will fly.

Let's Talk Communication

It may not be what you say but the tone of your voice, the way you move, and the look on your face that will be understood. Since people with Alzheimer's disease don't always understand words, make sure your facial expression is relaxed and friendly and that your tone of voice conveys a friendly, helpful, respectful attitude. Much of your success in caring for a person with dementia is your ability to communicate effectively and to interpret what the person is communicating. Even if you no longer understand what he is saying, still respond as though you do. It's like when a toddler is learning how to talk. If you respond as though you don't understand, he becomes frustrated and keeps repeating himself until you do understand. It's human nature to want to be understood.

Positive Non-verbal Communication

- Be aware of your body language and send a positive message.

- Try a calm, gentle, matter-of-fact approach.

- Reduce background noise by talking to the person in a place that is free from distractions.

- Position yourself directly in front of him and make sure you have his attention before you start to speak. (Most people with dementia lose peripheral vision on the left side.)

• Touching a person on the shoulder or holding his hand may help him focus on what you are trying to communicate.

• Show the person what you want him to do by demonstrating.

• Praise non-verbally through hugs, a caring smile, or a pat on the back

• Try a hug and change the subject.

• Walk away and try again later with a different approach.

Positive Verbal Communication

• Speak slowly in a low-pitched voice.

• Enunciate your words.

• Begin your conversation socially.

• Use short, familiar words and simple sentences.

• Talk in a warm, easy-going, pleasant manner.

• Ask simple questions that require a yes/no answer.

• Listen carefully.

• Give positive instructions; avoid "don't," "can't," or negative commands.

• Avoid questions that require short-term memory, such as: "Did your son come to see you today?"

• Communicate using a person's long-term memory. For example, say, "I hear you have a wonderful son."

• Give simple instructions, focusing on one task at a time. (The simple task of brushing one's teeth contains eleven steps!)

- Keep talking to residents, even if they cannot talk back.

When You Don't Understand
What They Are Communicating

- Listen actively and carefully.

- Focus on a word or phrase that makes sense.

- Respond to the emotional tone of the statement, not the word.

- Stay calm and be patient.

- Ask family members about possible meanings for words, names, or phrases.

- Respond as though you understand.

Things Not to Do

- Don't argue with the person.

- Don't order the person around.

- Don't be condescending.

- Don't talk about people in front of them.

Persons with dementia can hear, think, and feel emotions! Do not talk over, through, or about them as if they are not there. Avoid whispering, because it arouses suspicion. Yelling into a person's ear who cannot hear very well will only upset or frighten him. It's more effective to talk in low tones, enunciate, and speak slowly. Now is the best time to observe their body language because if or when they lose their ability to communicate, you have already developed another way to understand them.

The person with dementia is frightened of making a mistake, los-
ing his/her train of thought, or not finding the correct word to
express his feelings or meaning. Conversation may come out as
a jumble of words. Sensitive caregivers can assist by supplying
words, finishing sentences, and listening carefully
for connections and clues, and of course helping the person
to talk as comfortably as possible for as long as possible.
                                                    —Moyra Jones

New-Found Way to Communicate

_____

_____

_____

_____

_____

_____

_____

_____

_____

_____

_____

_____

_____

_____

_____

_____

_____

_____

Find the Treasures

Every one of us has been given many treasures, gifts, and talents. Find out what this person's treasure is. What makes her feel valued? What is she good at? She may have been a "rock hound," an artist, or a dancer. One way to find the treasures is by asking questions that she can easily answer. For instance, you may not get an answer if you ask an open-ended question, such as "Where did you grow up?" Instead ask, "Did you grow up on a farm or in town?" "Do you like dogs or cats?" If she has difficulty answering from two choices, the next step is to ask questions that can be answered with a yes or no: "Do you like to work in the garden?"

Ways to Bring Light to a Person's Treasures

I heard you can fix about anything.

So you're a good fisherman. Have you caught lots of big fish?

I have this brown thumb. I wish it was green like yours.

I heard you loved to dance. Did you ballroom dance?

I heard you make a wonderful rhubarb pie. I bet your husband loves that!

When you constantly remind her of her treasures, you are giving her back her history, knowledge, and accomplishments. Not only are you reminding her who she is; you're also talking about subjects she knows a lot about, which might make it easier to communicate.

> *Angela would walk around the facility and take down pictures and carry them around. Management thought they would solve this problem by bolting all the pictures to the wall. We later found out that Angela enjoyed interior decorating. We understand now why she takes pictures off the wall. We missed her "treasure" and went to great lengths to stop her from enjoying her treasure. Find their treasures and give it back to them.*

Two ladies were visiting in the back yard and there was a shovel stuck in the ground not far away. One lady sighed and said, "That's as far as he got spading for a garden . . . the worms looked so good he went fishing."

New-Found Treasure and How to Give It Back

Quality Connections

Does this sound familiar? You are walking down the hall and encounter Joe. You pat Joe on the shoulder and you say as you continue to your destination, "Hi Joe. How are you today?" Joe cannot focus that quickly and has stopped his walking and is trying to figure out what happened. "Did someone hit me on the shoulder? Am I suppose to be someplace?"

Making a Quality Connection

- Stop. To make a quality connection, you must stop and be still.

- Touch the person lightly on the hand or arm and say his name.

- Make eye contact.

- Make the connection: "Good morning, Joe. You. . . . sure . . . look . . . handsome . . . today."

For those who are in wheelchairs it makes a huge difference to kneel down to their level. Slow down between words and stop asking, "How are you?" When you ask "How are you" you will either get a list of all the things bothering them, which could take fifteen minutes to resolve, or they have to reflect on how they really feel. Moments of joy will instantly happen if you break this habit.

47

Instead, compliment, compliment, compliment! "Joe, I love that hat on you." "Alice, you really look good in that color. Your cheeks look so rosy today." Now, Alice may really have messy hair and look a little distraught. But you are making her feel better and giving her a good thought. Compliment a person on his treasures. Making quality connections will help retain a person's dignity, make him feel respected and valued, and make him feel like he belongs. Imagine if everyone made quality connections. I guarantee that morale would go up, and complimenting others might become contagious.

> *After attending one of my seminars, a lady called and said she always asked Chip, "How are you?" and he usually responded with frustration because he wasn't able to communicate clearly anymore. Well today, he was looking out the window with the sun shining on his face, and she commented, "Does that sun feel warm?" He said "yes." Since she knew he grew up in Chicago, she said, "Does it remind you of Chicago?" He said "yes." "Can you see the kids playing out on the street?" He said "yes." "And can you smell the asphalt?" He said "yes." "Enjoy your day, Chip." Then she walked away and realized she had just created a moment of joy. What better gift to give, and in a matter of seconds!*

People with dementia who have difficulty communicating can usually still respond with "yes" and "no" far into the disease. When you learn how to change the way you ask a question so the person is able to respond with a yes or no, you have obtained a powerful tool.

> *Richard would walk up and down the halls repeating, "I'm hungry, I'm hungry, I'm hungry." I walked up to him and asked, "What do you like to eat?" He just replied, "I'm hungry, I'm hungry." Reminding myself of this tool, I said, "Do you like chicken?" He said "no." "Do you like warm chocolate chip cookies from*

the oven?" He said "yes." "Do you like roast with potatoes?" He said, "Ah hah." "Do you like noodles?" He said, "Could live without it." "Do you like carrots?" He said, "Oh yeah." The list went on and on, and by the end I knew exactly what he liked and didn't like. Amazingly, his answers became more detailed and clear as we continued our conversation. This tool works, so use it!

Making quality connections also means thinking about the environment when you make a connection. People with Alzheimer's disease have difficulty with depth perception. They do not see white on white. This means that if you are wearing a white uniform and are standing against a white wall, you may look like a head and hands floating in space. Scary! If you wear black, you may seem like a hole in the wall. Wear mid-range colors like purple, green, bright yellow, or deep pink, so they can see you. Make changes in the environment to adjust for loss of depth perception. When you see someone resisting sitting down on the toilet seat, look to see if you have a white toilet seat with an off-white floor. If so, she probably doesn't see the toilet. If you are doing a painting project with them and their canvas is white against a white wall, they may not see the canvas. If they don't eat their potatoes, noodles, or boiled eggs on a white plate, it may be because they don't see the food. You may have to purchase bright blue plates, since we don't have too many bright blue foods; or just pour gravy over the potatoes to give it contrasting color. These are simple changes that make a big difference!

It's not so much the destination that matters, but it's the road you take to get there.

— Jeanne Yordi

New-Found Quality Connection

Take Action!

If you see frustration in the face of the person with dementia, or if she is expressing anger, take action as though you will take care of it for her. "I would be upset too. I will talk to management about fixing it." You might have to take physical action and leave the room. Go get a drink of water or whatever it takes to be gone for a few minutes. Other answers might be: "I will talk to your son about that." "I will call your husband." "I will call the doctor and ask his opinion." Your answer should include a person she trusts or a person of authority, so she feels like you have taken her seriously. Act like you have everything under control (even if you don't). She shouldn't have to worry about a thing. Wouldn't you love to have that feeling someday? What goes around comes around. Start today.

> Don was in charge of a manufacturing company most of his life. He made frequent comments about how no one was working hard "around here." Don came to me and said something needed to be done about these lazy workers. I said I would get right on it. I didn't move with that statement, and he became quite angry with me. His wife explained that he had always been in charge of many people. After this understanding, we acted as if he were our boss and responded with, "I'll get that done, sir," and took action by walking out the nearest door. Because of

his short-term memory, we could walk back in
within seconds; he responded better when he saw us
take action.

Hallucinations/Delusions

For the person with Alzheimer's disease, her hallucinations are very real, and just saying, "Alice, there aren't any snakes in your bed." won't usually solve the problem. Again, take action!

> *Pearl was yelling, "There's a fire in the house!*
> *There's a fire in the house!" Our answer was, "I*
> *called 911 and got everyone out. Come with me, I'll*
> *take you to a safe place." Then we walked Pearl out-*
> *side. We validated her feelings and then talked about*
> *other subjects she was interested in, like cooking or*
> *the weather, to help get her mind off the hallucina-*
> *tion. Sometimes it worked, sometimes it didn't. We*
> *also needed to consider her history. Had she ever*
> *been in a fire?*

Getting Robbed

People with dementia can become very suspicious. Rightly so, since they can no longer find their keys, purse, glasses, or jewelry. If the person is living in a facility, she has every reason to claim she is robbed, because someone takes her dentures, glasses, and clothes. A person might walk in her room in the middle of the night. People with dementia lose abilities, and they also lose the skills they need to adapt to these lost abilities. This means that if something is wrong, someone else must be the culprit. When a person still lives at home, her caregiver is the main target: "You stole my money," "A man was here and took all of my jewelry" (that man was her son). To a person with dementia, strange people seem to be coming and going all the time, because they can't recognize anyone anymore.

Doris came into the room and stated, "I got robbed last night." Our answer was: "I will talk to management, and we will tighten security. That should not happen here." Of course, we did not actually go to management, but it was important to make her feel like we were there to help. It's amazing how quickly she let go of her concern. If we had said, "Oh, it will be all right," she would have looked for another person who would listen to her. Think of it . . . wouldn't you be angry if you told someone you got robbed, and he ignored you? Blame it on management and take action!

> *Do things differently until the person with dementia is comfortable.*
> —Moyra Jones

New-Found Way to Take Action

The Illusion of Choice

If we opened a person's closet door and asked, "What would you like to wear today?" she may not respond because there are too many clothes to choose from. Instead, pull out two outfits and ask, "Which one would you would like to wear, the blue one or the red one?" She still may not be able to make the decision, so give her a reason to choose one of the outfits. "I like the blue dress. It brings out your beautiful blue eyes." This is called an "illusion of choice." Another wonderful way to give an illusion of choice is to say, "How about I choose today, and you can choose tomorrow?"

We need to give people with dementia an illusion of control to help restore their dignity. If we are passing out snacks, ask, "Would you like a cookie?" instead of putting a cookie in front of them without saying a word. "Would you like to sit by the window?" instead of "sit here." If you are changing something in their environment, ask their opinion. We need to change the way we get people to do what we need them to do. In other words, make it seem like it is their idea. No one likes to be bossed around or overlooked, no matter what age he is.

> When the staff told Ray it was time to eat, he would usually refuse. But if they left the plate of food on the table next to him and walked away, the food would be gone when they came back.

Frank didn't usually want to go to bed at night when someone told him it was time to do so. So they asked him, "I wonder where your room is. Frank, can you help me find it? Is it this door? No. Is it this door? Hey, we found it." For some reason, once he was in his room, he was easy to get into bed. The hard part was getting him there. What a treasure this illusion of choice became! Staff were able to use this tactic over and over, so everyone involved had less stress and more success.

> *Little things mean everything.*
> — Samuel Johnson

New-Found Choice and How You Simplified It

_____
_____
_____
_____
_____
_____
_____
_____
_____
_____
_____
_____
_____
_____
_____
_____

Your Mood Affects Their Mood

You better believe it . . . your mood does affect the mood of people with dementia! If you're rushed, they are rushed. If you're upset, they are upset. If you're happy, they are happy. Basically you decide what kind of day it's going to be. Now, I'm not saying it's easy. We all have bad days; that's life! But I can say that you will save so much time and frustration if you find a way to put yourself in a good mood, even if you are having one of those days. The blessing in disguise is that it's easy to change their mood—into a good mood, of course.

> *People always say I have so much energy, and I do. When I started working as an activity director in an Alzheimer's facility, I took my energy with me. I would enter the building all bubbly and hyper, talking loud and fast, as I always do. I felt like I was doing my job if I kept the people busy all day long. Well, the first six months were difficult, to say the least. People were bouncing off the walls! Wherever I would go, they followed me. They weren't able to sit down and relax with me around. Luckily, I couldn't keep up the pace, and one day I said to them, "I need to take a break. I'll be back in twenty minutes. Relax and enjoy the peace and quiet." When I returned, almost everyone was still sitting, and it was quiet. Amazing! It's one of those tools I keep in my front pocket to use frequently.*

Another tool to help calm people down is to sing two slow songs at the end of each stimulating activity or if they seem anxious—songs like "Silvery Moon" and "I'm Forever Blowing Bubbles." When you carry relaxing tools, you will be able to perform magic.

> *It's difficult to think anything but pleasant thoughts while eating a home-grown tomato.*
> — Lewis Grizzard

New-Found Treasure That Makes You Happy

Look Good, Feel Good, Play Good

Isn't this statement true for whatever you are doing, whether it is sports, interviewing for a job, going to church, going out to dinner, meeting with friends? The opposite is also true. When we don't look good, we usually stay in the comforts of our home so no one will see us. This concept applies to all human beings. Imagine if someone put a purple shirt on you and pants, but you really prefer dresses. Maybe all your clothes are too tight or have rips in them. How would you feel about socializing with others now?

What we wear affects our mood. Why is it that when a person gets old we think it is OK not to look good? Every morning, try to be patient and allow ample time for a person to get ready for the day (comb hair, shave, lotion hands, apply cologne, apply lipstick, and put on clothes he or she feels good wearing). So what if he eats breakfast in his pajamas or eats breakfast a little later? Don't we enjoy the mornings when we get to putter around? Make it a priority to take the time to help the person with dementia to look good, so he feels good and then will play good (function higher). Your day will be better, too.

> *Sarah loved to wear red and chose to wear red every day. On the days that her red outfits were in the laundry, she had a green outfit. I swear she wasn't as congenial when she wore green. But on the days she wore red, she looked good and felt good, so she*

received more compliments. "Sarah, I sure like red on you." She replied proudly, "I do, too. My mother never let me wear it because she said it was the devil's color, but I like it." We knew a bit about her past, and she had not been very close to her mother, and she had been the tomboy of the family. Seldom did she talk about her mother, except when she was rebelling. So this becomes a wonderful story, a story we all can relate to. She should wear red every day.

Compliment, compliment, compliment! Compliment the person on the attributes that she likes about herself. Clothing is one way we express who we are and what our personality is. We are all wonderfully different; give people opportunities to express individual qualities.

There was a dynamic-looking lady in a care facility. She had on a striking pink dress, pink lipstick, pink cheeks, pink fingernails, white purse, and white pumps. Her hair was every bit in place, and she walked with confidence. Because of her short-term memory loss and because this was her favorite dress, she didn't remember what she wore the day before, so she would always pick out the same dress. Staff had a real problem with someone wearing the same dress seven days a week. They also had a difficult time getting the dress off the lady to get it washed. Their solution was to pour coffee on it, so she would have to take it off. If you think this story sounds horrifying, you are absolutely right. This dress made the lady look good, feel good, and play good. She dressed to the hilt all by herself, because this dress was familiar, and it triggered the experience of the total glamorous process. Of course, the dress needed to be cleaned every once in a while, but the answer isn't to damage it or tell the lady that she smells. Think how insulted you would be if someone told you that. If you think about her personality and body language, a better answer might be, "There is a

*handsome man visiting tonight. Let me wash your
dress so you will look wonderful tonight." It also
helps to buy six of the same outfit that she likes to
wear and six pairs of the same shoes that she likes.*

If you are a caregiver at home, this is one area where
outside assistance is a good idea. Ask a family member to
help or hire someone to get your loved one bathed and
dressed each morning. You can have a quiet hour to yourself, and then the two of you can start your day together,
refreshed and ready to go.

*Puttering is really a time to be alone, to dream and to get
in touch with yourself. . . . To putter is to discover.*
—Alexandra Stoddard

New-Found Favorite Clothes, Shoes, Hairstyle

_____

_____

_____

_____

_____

_____

_____

_____

_____

_____

_____

_____

_____

_____

_____

_____

_____

_____

_____

_____

_____

_____

_____

_____

_____

_____

_____

_____

_____

_____

_____

_____

_____

_____

_____

_____

_____

_____

_____

_____

_____

_____

The Power of Touch

Touch can reach through the fog and fear of people with dementia. It is a basic need of life. Touch begins before we are born—a pregnant woman massages her stomach, and the infant perceives this. This need continues until the last breath of life leaves our body. Touch can be simple and spontaneous, such as a handshake or a pat on the back. Touch can be deeper and more complicated, like a massage or dancing. Research shows that gentle massaging can ease tension and anxiety. In addition, regularly touching individuals and allowing ourselves to be touched can create a bond with a person who has lost the ability to speak. It is important to remember, however, that not everyone likes to be touched.

Suggestions When Touching

- Begin gradually; be sensitive to the person's reaction.

- Treat the person with respect. Ask before touching.

- Make sure the person is aware of your presence before you touch him.

- Offer touch from non-humans, like dogs and cats.

Dawn Nelson claims that "touch can help 'ground' those who are spatially disoriented, helping to bring such people back to their bodies and increase their awareness in present space and time." In the latest stage of Alzheimer's, touch might be the most powerful gift you can give. Sometimes a warm embrace is more healing than any wonder drug. Look for those situations when you shouldn't say a word but just reach out and hold a loved one.

Each of us are like angels with only one wing—
we can fly only by embracing another.
                                        —Barbara Johnson

New-Found Positive Way to Touch

_____

_____

_____

_____

_____

_____

_____

_____

_____

_____

_____

_____

_____

_____

_____

_____

Kick Starting

When people have Alzheimer's, they usually lose the ability to start a motion and to locate certain parts of the body. We need to "kick start" them. In other words, if a person is sitting down for a meal and not eating, one reason may be because he cannot start the motion. Place your hand over his hand and assist with two bites. He might then start eating on his own.

If you ask him to put on his sock, but he doesn't respond, touch his foot and cue him again to put on his sock. It doesn't matter what the task is—if he responds blankly, start the motion and touch that part of his body to get him started.

> *One of my favorite things to do was give everyone lotion and encourage hand massages. When I asked Edith if she would like some lotion, she would nod her head and then just sit there with a dab of lotion on her hand. I put her hands together and helped her rub in the lotion. After a short time she started doing it on her own.*

Another way to help a person understand what you want him to do is to demonstrate the motion, like brushing his teeth or putting on clothes. Another method is cueing, which means to explain one task at a time as briefly and simply as possible. Your goal is to help the person stay independent as long as possible. If the person is struggling, just help him with the task and let him try again the next day. People with Alzheimer's have good and bad days, just like us.

Avoid helping too much. If you try to do everything for them, they may become more dependent on you, making it more work in the long run. Most importantly, allow them more time to accomplish each task.

A care provider was trying to get a gentleman to take out his dentures. This had become a daily struggle. Finally, she pulled out her dentures to demonstrate what she wanted him to do. It worked! He took out his dentures.

A care provider was struggling to put a diaper on a lady. So she showed her what she wanted by putting one on herself. It worked! The lady not only cooperated, but her attitude changed about wearing a Depend.

When Mr. Evans came into the Alzheimer's facility, he functioned at a pretty high level. He was still able to do accounting-like work in the afternoon. I took maternity leave for about four months. When I returned, he was in a wheelchair and had declined rapidly. I asked the staff what had happened. One staff member said she wasn't sure, but now whenever she asks him to brush his teeth, he just opens his mouth. I realize that I didn't witness the decline, but the fact that he just opened his mouth, making no attempt to brush his own teeth, told me staff was doing too much for him, making him dependent on others.

Attitude

God guides my hand and
shows me again and again
how to hold the brush.
Yet each day He lets me choose the colors with which
I paint the canvas of my mind.

—Teresa Burleson

New-Found Area to Kick Start

_____

_____

_____

_____

_____

_____

_____

_____

_____

_____

_____

_____

_____

_____

_____

_____

_____

_____

Memory-Enhanced Environments

*Don't wait for the roses,
stop and smell the daisies.*

Trigger Fond Memories

Our five senses are the closest connection to our memory. When you *smell* cinnamon rolls, you think about the cinnamon rolls Grandma made. When I *say*, "I'd lose my head if it wasn't attached," I think of my mother, who said it often when she couldn't find something. When you *see* a certain flower, you may think about a certain person. When you *hear* the train whistle, you remember running beside the train waving at the conductor. When you *feel* a silky pink fabric, you think about a favorite dress.

Realistically, we can no longer ask a person with Alzheimer's to make a casserole, but she can wash off vegetables, taste different foods, talk about favorite meals, and hear a prayer before she eats. All of these things will trigger her long-term memory. When we surround her with things that trigger her five senses, we are ultimately triggering her long-term memory.

Joan and Ray had met at a singles group. Ray asked her what she thought of the group. Joan replied, "There's just a bunch of losers here." Not long after that, they started dating and eventually got married. So faithfully twice a year Ray sent her a dozen roses with a note that said, "From the loser." Ray was diagnosed with Alzheimer's before the age of fifty-two. Joan kept him at home for a long time. They would go grocery shopping together, and one day Ray wandered off. When she found him, he was in the flower department. She asked what he was doing, and he stated, "Want buy." "You want to buy some roses?" she asked. He nodded. He wasn't able to figure out how to pay for the roses, so Joan bought them. They took the roses home and put them in the vase. The next morning he walked into the kitchen and asked about the roses. She said, "You bought them for me last night, remember?" She saw a light in his eye, and he replied, "Oh yeah, they are from the loser." She cried. Moments later he was "gone" again. But she opened the window to his memory for a moment.

A facility would have tea parties. When the ladies saw the tea set and smelled the tea, they would sit up straighter, point out their pinkie fingers, and socialize with one another. They were given an experience to trigger their memory on how to act at tea parties.

A gentleman who had Parkinson's disease went into a comatose state, and many different methods of therapy were being tried. The most effective therapy was to constantly remind him in conversation and through touch who he was. He had been a basketball coach most of his life and loved the game. His therapy was to address him as "coach," talk basketball with him, and put his hands on a basketball. The family said this is the therapy that "brought him back."

Pictures from the past can trigger memories. Placing items that are special for that person in his room triggers memories. If he is in bed most of the time, we can place things outside his window that he would enjoy looking at: a dog house (no need for the dog if you wish), bird feeders, small windmills, bird houses, fake animal figures, flower or vegetable garden, hanging plant, old bicycle, tractor, the American flag (yes! yes!)—the list goes on.

Another way to trigger memories is through our conversations. Conversations about outhouses, wood stoves, first radios, first kiss, holiday traditions, wedding day, raising children, the first dollar he earned, or memories of his parents. When we talk about subjects from his childhood, memories trickle out. When he can no longer verbally communicate, we can still give him back his childhood memories. If you don't know about his childhood memories, share one of yours!

> *For the sense of smell, almost more than any other,*
> *has the power to recall memories*
> *and it is a pity that we use it so little.*
> — Rachel Carson

New-Found Memories and How to Trigger Them

_____

_____

_____

_____

_____

_____

_____

_____

_____

_____

_____

_____

_____

Create a Safe Haven

If someone came into your home and took all the items that are significant to you, would you want to live there? Would you still find pleasure and enjoyment being in your home? The things you choose to have in your home make it your safe haven, because you are surrounded by things that bring you comfort.

Who is this person you are caring for? What are her hobbies, favorite pastimes? What brings her joy? What items is she familiar with? By filling her life with what makes her a unique individual, memories will flow when she enters her room, because it is filled with things she loves and recognizes. For instance, if an individual loved to fish, you might place pictures of fish on the wall, bring in fishing poles and a fishing net, and place a tackle box in the corner with fishing lures (hooks removed), string, etc. For a person who loved to make quilts, place a beautiful quilt on her bed or on the wall, put together a pretty sewing box with string, fabric pieces, pin cushion (without pins), safe scissors, pattern books, and measuring tape. If there is room, find a place for an old sewing machine that doesn't work. If the person lives in a facility, accept the fact that what you bring in might get lost, broken, or found in someone else's room; twenty residents have twenty rooms. Be sure to "gift" or donate the items. Also realize you will probably create moments for other people, because they might love to fish and sew, too. Be realistic, and constantly ask yourself what the person is able to use safely. She can no longer make a quilt, but she can still feel fabrics, cut out shapes, look at patterns, and talk about the memories this experience triggers. That's a treasure!

> *A lady moved into a facility, and she explained how she hadn't moved in yet. She actually was moved in except for her favorite chair, and that was how she expressed that something significant in her life was missing.*

Make the person's room look, feel, and smell of individuality. We do sometimes make the mistake of buying all new decorations and wardrobe, and the room becomes someone else's, because nothing is familiar. Decorate with items that define who this person is, so when anyone enters her room, he sees a unique human being and instantly knows something valuable about this person.

Place decorations five feet high and below, so she is able to see and appreciate her belongings. If she is in a wheelchair, lower decorations to that height. Please remember that wheelchairs are for transfer—they do not offer any type of comfort. Your loved one's favorite chair offers comfort. Her own bed and bedroom furniture offer comfort. Her treasured possessions offer comfort. The more comfortable she is, the more content she will be.

> *A gentleman who had been in the army would wake up in the morning thinking he was in an army barracks because his room didn't have much more than two beds. Being in the army didn't trigger fond memories, so this environment may have caused a level of fear. You could also get this person to stand straight up and march by saying, "Attention! March!"*

> *We cannot give them their memory back,*
> *but we can give them an experience that triggers memory.*
> — Moyra Jones

New-Found Treasures That Bring Comfort

Life Reflection

Look around your home. Do you see pictures to remind you of special times? If other people look at those pictures, they just see people. You look at those pictures, and you see a wonderful story behind each one.

Every person should have pictures around him that reflect his adventures in life. One way to do this is to create a life panel or a life story book. A life panel or story book includes pictures from a person's past and significant information about him. Collect photocopies of pictures of him when he was younger: wedding picture, school picture, baby picture, family picture, etc. The reason you want to photocopy pictures is because the pictures may get lost or damaged. It is difficult to replace an original but easy to replace a photocopy.

Include pictures of people who are significant in that person's life and then write under each picture the names of the people in the picture and their relationship. Write a short biography and add any information that may be significant to the person: pets, hobbies, past occupation, personality, things to talk about or not to talk about. Place these pictures neatly on mat board or cork board or in a photo album. If you want to hang up pictures of the person's wedding day or graduation picture, one way is to have the picture enlarged, photocopied, and put in a pretty frame with a description. There is little visible difference between an original picture and one that is copied. Then hang the life panel and pictures on a wall in his room, so when people enter his room they can make a "quality connection." Instantly they see a person with history, family, friends, and life.

I hear story after story about how pictures get torn down—like that fiftieth anniversary picture, pictures taken last week, or the Polaroid picture hanging outside his room. This is because what we think he is seeing is someone else with his spouse; or he doesn't know why a picture of someone else is hanging in or near his room. Again this hints to us that he thinks he is younger than he really is, so the pictures that are most useful are the ones taken from his youth.

It can be helpful to place a picture of the person, when he was young, outside his room. This enables him to distinguish his door from all the other doors, especially if he lives in a facility. Above all, enjoy digging into your history and finding out more about the one you love.

> *Pat loved to fish in her younger years, and that was something to be proud of in her day. She had a picture of herself holding a thirty-pound salmon on a distinguished-looking dock. This picture was hung right outside her room, and when anyone entered the facility, she would show them the picture and talk about how big the fish was. When Pat could no longer communicate very well, she would point at the picture and nod her head, and her eyes showed you how proud she was of that day. Her room was also decorated very beautifully, and the other ladies enjoyed being in her room, too.*

When we bring sunshine into the lives of others, we are warmed by it ourselves.

—Barbara Johnson

New-Found Picture and Who Is in the Picture

_____
_____
_____
_____
_____
_____
_____
_____
_____
_____
_____
_____
_____
_____
_____
_____
_____
_____
_____
_____
_____
_____
_____
_____
_____
_____
_____

Replacing Priceless Treasures

What looks like junk to you may be a priceless treasure to someone full of fond memories. She should not be robbed of these treasures. If there is something of monetary value, like a tea set, jewelry, wallet, purse, or rock collection, replace it with something that resembles the real item.

> Mary was in tears, and I asked her why she was crying. She pointed at my wedding ring, and in jumbled words she expressed how her husband would be upset when he found out she had lost her wedding ring. Her husband was no longer living, and her family took her ring, but she could not remember that.

There are many ways to replace what is missing. Wedding rings have a priceless value, so replace the ring with a fake one. Wallets and purses need to be replaced as well, but be sure to have ten purses and wallets in the closet for backup in case the original gets lost. Imagine not having your wallet or purse with you. You would feel a little insecure, too. This is why many people with dementia living in a facility say they cannot stay for dinner—because they don't have any money to pay for it. I understand the hassle of accepting money and trying to give it back. An easier answer might be to tell the person his spouse paid for his meal, or use fake money. Men especially should have a little change in their pocket or a few dollars in their wallet so they feel they are able to pay if they need to. Men also like such items as membership cards, AAA card, business cards, and receipts. Women, on the other hand, are happy with a comb, handkerchief, pictures, etc. Be sure to enclose a card with the person's present address in case he or she becomes lost.

Another wonderful safety measure is to sign them up with the Safe Return Program at the nearest office of the Alzheimer's Association. This enables the community to help bring them home safely. These people are priceless treasures, too.

> *We too often love things and use people, when we should be using things and loving people.*
> —Unknown

New-Found Treasures You Replaced

_____

_____

_____

_____

_____

_____

_____

_____

_____

_____

_____

_____

_____

_____

Fill Habits of a Lifetime

We all have habits of a lifetime. It could be going to bed at 12:00 and getting up at 8:00. It could be sleeping with a feather pillow, eating popcorn at night to relax, or always taking a shower in the morning. For one woman I knew, it was eating a cheese sandwich and hot water for breakfast, and in another case it was never eating breakfast. Once we know that the person has always done things a certain way, it should be accepted. When we don't know, we assume something is wrong with the person who sleeps in until 10:00 or does not eat breakfast.

When someone has Alzheimer's, it is very difficult for him to tell us what his habits of a lifetime are. Grasp the moment now and write down your own habits of a lifetime if you want quality care when you get older. If you ever lose the ability to communicate, someone else will decide what your wants and wishes are. Keep a journal throughout your life so you create a window for others to see inside.

The staff told me about a belligerent man who was still cognitive but very uncooperative. I knocked on his door and walked into his room at about 9:00 at night. The room was very warm, he was resting on top of his covers with his day clothes on, and there were pictures of horses all over his room. I explained I was just visiting and asked him about the pictures of horses on the wall. He eagerly told me how he was

*a Texas ranger and rode all over the United States to
compete in rodeos. We had a delightful conversation
about him sleeping under the stars and being a
bachelor all of his life roaming the countryside.*

*When I left the room, I thought about our con-
versation. He sleeps on top of his covers with his
clothes on because he is accustomed to sleeping under the stars, and his room is really warm because he
is used to the Texas heat. Since he never married,
taking orders from staff, who were predominantly
women, probably was difficult for him. In addition,
if he did not have pictures of horses around him, he
would essentially lose his sense of identity. With
this new information, I was able to understand him;
and more importantly, this was an opportunity to
write down his habits of a lifetime while he was still
able to tell us. Just imagine how aggressive he could
be if we tried to put him in pajamas and tuck him
into bed!*

*The staff talked about a gentleman whom they
would put into bed, and within minutes he was up
wandering around again. They spoke to his wife and
asked what his evening routine was, because maybe
they were missing something. They explained how
they would have a snack and then put him in his
pajamas and tuck him into bed. The wife said he
never wore pajamas, he always slept in the nude.
Putting pajamas—clothing—on him might have
meant that it was time to get up and start the day.*

*The less we interfere with a person's lifestyle the easier it is for
them to adapt to new surroundings.*
                                        —Chaplain R.A. Wilcox

New-Found Habits of a Lifetime

_____

_____

_____

_____

_____

_____

_____

_____

_____

_____

_____

_____

_____

_____

_____

_____

_____

_____

_____

_____

_____

_____

_____

_____

_____

_____

_____

Music Does Wonders

Even if a person is unable to communicate clearly, she can still sing a familiar song if we "kick start" the song. This kick starting also applies to people who don't have Alzheimer's. If I asked you to sing "Top of the World," could you? Probably not, unless you are a big fan of Karen Carpenter. But if I started singing, "I'm on top of the world, looking down on creation and the only explanation I can find . . . ," if you hear the melody with the words together, you probably would be able to sing right along with me.

The same works with a person who has dementia. I can almost guarantee that if you started singing "Jesus Loves Me" to a person in the late stages of Alzheimer's, you would see some sort of positive response, which could be as simple as comfort in her eyes. And what a gift comfort is! Music is therapy, and the results are amazing!

Dorothy usually just shuffled around mumbling noises to herself, but when someone started singing "I've been working on the railroad," she piped right up and sang every word. When she was singing, she shuffled less and sometimes stood up straighter, and you could see the enjoyment in her face. When staff wanted Doris to cooperate in situations in which she was usually very disagreeable, singing this song usually helped.

*When I was an activity director, we would sing for
an hour over shift change every afternoon, which is
usually the most difficult time of the day. While we
sang, people navigated toward the living room and
joined in on their own. Shift change became less stressful because the residents were less aware of staff coming and going. The common problem of "I want to go
home" was reduced, and music almost always lifted
people's spirits, staff and residents alike.*

If you play music on the radio, be sure it is an "oldies"
station. I highly recommend getting tapes from the 1900s to
1940s. For a person with dementia, voices on the radio
might seem like someone is actually talking to him, and he
doesn't know where the voices are coming from. The look
of radios today is unfamiliar, so it helps to buy a replica of
an earlier model, just to trigger memories. Don't be afraid
to play the big band peppy music, classical music, or other
types of music—just be sure that you end with a soothing, familiar song. Depending on the task, avoid playing music
while asking the person to do a task. For example, don't play
music while trying to have a conversation, playing a game,
or eating dinner. Although it is usually fine to play soothing
music before meals to help a person relax, during the meal
it is better to turn the music off. It is difficult for some
people to eat, let alone eat with noise in the background.
Again, use your experience to help make these decisions. If
it works, it works. If it doesn't, it doesn't.

The myth about people with dementia having difficulty
doing the same thing for a long period of time is not always
true. If they like what they are doing and are familiar with
the task, they can do the same thing for a long time. So
don't be afraid to sing every day for a full hour. Everyone
loves music, and music triggers good feelings.

Keep on Singing
*Like any good mother, when Karen found out that
another baby was on the way, she helped her three-
year-old son, Michael, prepare for the new sibling.*

Day after day, Michael sang to his sister in Mommy's tummy, building a bond of love with his little sister before he even met her.

In time, the labor pains began. Serious complications arose during delivery and after a long struggle, Michael's sister was born. She was in very serious condition and flown to a hospital nearby. The pediatrician had to tell the parents, "There is very little hope. Be prepared for the worst." Michael, however, kept begging his parents to let him see his sister. "I want to sing to her," he kept saying, but kids are never allowed in intensive care. Karen made up her mind, and she decided to take Michael whether they liked it or not. The head nurse saw him and bellowed, "Get that kid out of here now!" Karen rose up strong, and she looked right into the nurse's face and stated, "He is not leaving until he sings to his sister!"

Michael gazed at the tiny infant losing the battle to live. After a moment, he began to sing in the pure-hearted voice of a three-year-old, "You are my sunshine, my only sunshine, you make me happy when skies are gray . . ." Instantly the baby girl seemed to respond. The pulse rate began to calm down and become steady. "Keep on singing, Michael," encouraged his mother with tears in her eyes. "You never know, dear, how much I love you, Please don't take my sunshine away." As Michael sang to his sister, the baby's ragged, strained breathing became as smooth as a kitten's purr. "Keep on singing, sweetheart!" "The other night, dear, as I lay sleeping, I dreamed I held you in my arms . . ." Michael's little sister began to relax, as rest, healing rest, seemed to sweep over her. "Keep on singing, Michael." Karen glowed. "You are my sunshine, my only sunshine. Please don't take my sunshine away . . ."

The next day, the very next day, the little girl was well enough to go home! Woman's Day maga-

zine called it "The Miracle of a Brother's Song."
The medical staff just called it a miracle. Karen
called it a miracle of God's love!

Never give up on the people you love.
Love is so incredibly powerful.

New-Found Favorite Songs

_____ ___

_____

_____

_____

_____

_____

_____

_____

_____

_____

_____

_____

_____

_____

_____

_____

_____

_____

_____

A Commercial about TV

TV can have negative effects that we blame on Alzheimer's but is actually a result of watching TV. The content should not be violent or involve everyday life situations, because people with dementia cannot separate themselves from what is happening on TV. If someone got shot on TV, the person with dementia might think someone really got shot. Choose TV programs with happy positive content, like musicals, Shirley Temple movies, Lawrence Welk, movies about animals or babies, sports, and possibly some game shows (but you better have prizes in the mail). Even *I Love Lucy* has a story line too detailed to follow and is likely to lose the person's interest.

Story told by many: My mother called me and said she didn't know how she was going to feed all these people in her house, and asked if I could come over to help her. I went over to her house, and no one was there, but the TV was on. All those people she was seeing were on TV.

A gentleman was telling his wife about how the place he lived in was dealing drugs. He said drugs were being brought in on the food truck so no one would notice. He was very concerned and wanted his wife to call the police. She went along with his story and said she would take care of it. The next day she met a friend of hers for lunch, and her friend told her about a show she watched the night before about drug dealers smuggling drugs in on food trucks. What is happening on TV is happening to a person with dementia.

There are days when any electrical appliance in the house, including the vacuum cleaner, seems to offer more enter-tainment possibilities than the TV set.

—Harriet Van Horne

New-Found Entertainment

_____
_____
_____
_____
_____
_____
_____
_____
_____
_____
_____
_____
_____
_____
_____
_____
_____
_____
_____

Where's the Outhouse?

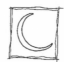

When incontinence begins to occur, first check the environment to see whether you are making it easy for the person to find the bathroom. One reason people with dementia become incontinent is because they can't remember where the bathroom is located. Verbal reminders alone are not enough because of their short-term memory loss. Changes in the environment can make all the difference.

Suggested Changes

- Have a night light on in the bathroom. People with dementia walk where they are able to see.

- Leave the bathroom door open so they can see the toilet. They need to see the toilet to know that that is the bathroom.

- Replace the toilet seat with a brown or mid-range colored seat to distinguish the toilet seat from the floor.

- Paint the wall behind the toilet a mid-range color so the toilet stands out from the wall.

- Place a large three-D picture of a toilet on the outside of the door 5' or lower.

- Paint a half moon (outhouse symbol) on the door.

- Paint the bathroom door a different color from other doors. Then you can easily say, "It is the red door over there."

- Place the toilet paper in direct view.

Also try using different bathroom terms, such as "out-house," "privy," or "lavatory." Your loved one may never have called it "toilet" or "bathroom," so she doesn't understand what you are saying. *Avoid* asking if she needs to go to the bathroom, because she will naturally say no.

While in the bathroom, practice being quiet and invisible by placing yourself to the side or behind the person. Figure out what her habit of a lifetime or routine is when using the bathroom. Organize a routine so you know when to discreetly remind her it's time to use the bathroom. Placing your hand lightly on her shoulder may stop her from getting up and down. Above all, never use restraints, and always reassure.

To affect the quality of the day, that is the highest of arts.
— Henry David Thoreau

New-Found Bathroom Routine and
What You Call "the Bathroom"

_____

_____

_____

_____

_____

_____

_____

_____

It's Saturday Night! Bath Time!

Motivate, motivate, motivate! Whatever you are having difficulty getting a person with dementia to do, be creative and think of a way so he will want to do it. The issue of taking a shower is a big one for those with Alzheimer's, and I will address it thoroughly, so that you understand their distress, yet give you solutions to make bath time bearable.

One reason showers are so stressful is because they are unfamiliar. When this person was growing up, he probably took baths, not showers. Perhaps he didn't have running water, so the noise from the water can be alarming. He usually washed his hair in the sink, so shampooing his hair in the shower, with water running over his eyes, is an unfamiliar process. If he has a hearing loss and there is a lot of noise in the bathroom (fan, water running, people talking, etc.), it can be very confusing. Since he can't hear you, it is difficult to understand what your purpose is. He may not be able to see the water running down his arm, so he could perceive it to feel like bugs. There may be a definite justifiable fear of water from a past experience, but he is unable to communicate as such. It might just feel and look cold in the bathroom (stark, hard, white tiled walls).

People of that generation tend to be extremely private people, and your loved one may have dressed in the closet. Victims of the Holocaust might think they are in a gas chamber. Being naked may trigger memories of being molested.

I know these aren't pleasant reasons why they don't like showers, but the point is to stop blaming the reactions that occur solely on the disease. When we say a person with dementia does something because of the disease, we are essentially giving up on one valuable question: "Why?" Why is he reacting like he does? The key is to explore the family bathing practices. Once we know why, we either will understand and accept, or we will take the first step to figure out a solution to create change. The goal is to prevent or at least lessen the fear of bathing.

Preserving Modesty

- Sew two towels at the top corners, creating a poncho to put over the person while in the shower, or just put a towel over his lap. When the towels are wet, use them to clean him off. Have a dry poncho ready to put on after the shower/bath to dry him off.

- Don't hover over him. If possible, do something else while he is bathing: clean, read a book, or pretend you are looking for something (quietly).

- Acknowledge that you respect his privacy by telling him so or looking away when possible.

- Acknowledge his feelings and use genuine magic words. "I am here if you need me." "I understand, we will take it slow, and I will be careful." "Can I help with that?"

- Show the person you do care with assuring words, positive body language, and a genuine tone of voice.

- Start the bathing process by washing safe, less intimidating areas, such as feet and arms.

Helpful Bath Tub Hints

- If the person is still mobile, I recommend regular baths. Fill the tub one-third full before the person is in the room to avoid her being bothered by the noise.

- For some people, bubbles and soft music help them relax.

- Be sure to place a mid-range colored towel over the seat or at the bottom of the tub so the person sees where to sit and the seat is no longer cold. (See page 49 for information on color and perception.)

- Make the bathroom look, feel, and smell like a bathroom with pretty towels and a colorful shower curtain.

- Increase the light level three times, so the person doesn't feel like she is in a darkened room.

- Give the person control by letting her have her own "stuff" (washcloth, soap, glass).

Helpful Shower Hints

- Do say "wash up" or "clean up" instead of the word "shower."

- Instead of shower heads, use a colored pail with two colored glasses and have the person help scoop the water out, so he sees what is going to happen and can relate this to the familiar sponge bath.

- Use step-by-step instructions and bathe slowly.

Helpful Environmental Hints

- Reduce noise, rush, and glare.
- Paint the walls a warm soothing color.

- Use solid midrange colored towels, which look warmer and can be seen against white walls.

- Keep the bathroom really, really warm. We know the person already feels cold, and it's difficult to enjoy anything when you are cold.

More Helpful Hints

- Give simple step-by-step instructions and tasks.

- Focus all your attention on the person.

- Touch gently. Older people's skin becomes paper thin and very sensitive. Washing with a wash cloth or using a strong spray of water may hurt. Use soft towels.

- Bribe with a favorite treat. It's hard to be combative with a cookie in each hand. "After you take a shower I will get you a big bowl of ice cream."

- Motivate: "Let's get freshened up. It will feel good."

- With a businessman, make an appointment on paper and have him sign his name.

- If the person absolutely resists, leave and try again later.

- Find out the person's habit of a lifetime concerning showers (Did he take a shower in the morning or evening? Did he use a soap bar or wash cloth? What was the water temperature?).

- Give a reason why the person should get cleaned up—for example, someone is visiting or there is church the next day.

- Find ways to give an illusion of control.

- Stick to a routine!

- "It's Saturday night! You get to be the first to take a bath. The water is so warm!" (And note that every night can be Saturday night!)

- Make a verbal and written date on their calendar.

George didn't want to take a shower, and it had been two weeks since his last shower. Staff was at their wits' end with finding a solution, so one of the staff called George on the phone and acted like his wife. She told him they were going to visit friends tonight, and he better get cleaned up. It worked! He took a shower. The next time a better answer might be to have the wife really call and tell him something that will encourage him to get cleaned up. He is less likely to hit you if he understands the reason why he needs to get cleaned up.

As they were lowering Therstin into a Jacuzzi he yelled "Pig! Pig!" He was a farmer and thought they were lowering him into boiling water. This is how they would get the skin off pigs.

A lady being encouraged to get into a Jacuzzi stated with much resistance, "I don't want soup! I don't want soup!" The large Jacuzzi was a big pot of boiling soup.

Avoid Jacuzzis with a person who has dementia. For a person who is not cognitively impaired, a Jacuzzi can be very therapeutic.

Another important point to realize is that this person is having partial showers all through the week. Her hair gets washed at the beauty salon, and we clean her private areas if she is incontinent. All we have left are the legs, chest, and arms, which may be easily done with a traditional sponge bath. Don't feel like you have to submerge a person in water to get her clean.

If you work in a facility, try having shower experts. This

means choosing staff who are good at giving showers and whose main job is to give showers. This not only creates a familiar shower routine for each resident but seeing a familiar face is comforting. Creating a routine is a powerful tool! The shower experts truly become experts at what they do. Priceless!

> *A friend of mine told me she was the only one who was able to get this lady to take a shower. I said "How do you do it?" She said, "I really like this lady, and others don't because she can be difficult but I say to her, 'June, if you let me help with your shower I promise to make you beautiful.' And I do make her beautiful by combing her hair and putting on her favorite dress. It's quite simple."*

It can be that simple! If you are genuine and show the person you care, they will be more likely to cooperate with you. There is a saying I call having "IT." "IT" is a gift that comes naturally. Some of us are naturally wonderful working with older people. Some of us are naturally wonderful with children. Find your strength and focus on it. You will do amazing things!

> *Life is either a daring adventure or nothing. To keep our faces toward change and behave like free spirits in the presence of fate is strength undefeatable.*
>
> — Helen Keller

New-Found Bath Time Routine

_____

_____

_____

_____

_____

_____

Enhanced Moments

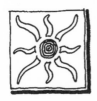

Touch many . . .
radiate your warmth.

Simple Pleasures

Think back to when you were a child and of all the simple pleasures you found: watching ants build their house, lying under the stars, running out in the rain, licking a lollipop, eating ice cream, walking through tall grass, finding a new flower, searching for beautiful rocks—simple pleasures we need to relive again.

A simple pleasure for an older person might be one of those things; it might be having her hair combed slowly, getting a back rub, getting lotion rubbed into her hands, receiving flowers, having someone gently brush her teeth, eating with a friend—the list is endless.

Focus on simple pleasures. It's not spending hours organizing a big party or buying the person a whole new wardrobe. It's all about fulfilling basic needs to the fullest. It's as simple as cleaning someone's glasses. You will be amazed by the gratitude you receive because she can see better. It's truly a gift, especially in the last stages of Alzheimer's, to understand the importance of simple pleasures.

This is a story my grandma wrote while in a nursing home watching a bird outside her window. In the beginning it doesn't make perfect sense, but read on, because it is a beautiful story. You will hear so much more if you take the time to listen to a person with dementia.

No one would think I have to see my articles to write and I studied long to find something to write about. Then about a block away a drama took place way up in a tall tree . . . "Unheard Chirp" by Nellie Larson. Two birds appeared, both looking very tired. The older bird started nest building while little Peter sat in another tree feeling very neglected. But mother was so busy building it didn't matter. At last the nest was finished and the mother bird laid an egg. The nest was lined with the soft down of her breast. Day after day she sat. It seemed such a long time. Each day she turned the egg. At last she heard a peep and a tiny hole appeared. Then a bigger one. Mother helped and soon the little fellow was out and drying nicely. Mother was so proud of him as he dried and turned a nice yellow, soft down. The End.

When you get older, joy is . . . birds, flower beds and young people.
—Bruce and Rhea Fletcher

New-Found Simple Pleasure

_____

_____

_____

_____

_____

_____

_____

_____

_____

_____

You've Got Mail!

Everyone has a lifetime of getting the mail. Who would you be without your mail? It's a way of daily connecting with the outside world and knowing what is going on around you. Even if you feel uncomfortable visiting someone with Alzheimer's, a wonderful gift you can always give is mail. Send a magazine subscription to him on a subject he enjoys! Since people with dementia usually lose the ability to read, find magazines with lots of distinct clear pictures.

We all love to receive packages in the mail, so send thoughtful, simple gifts, such as pretty jewelry, candy, poems, perfume, fishing lures, or fun things. A facility can "create" mail by recycling unwanted junk mail, magazines, or newspapers. If you live near a small town, order the community newspaper. I don't recommend subscribing to a city paper, which probably has bad news. Today's news can be extremely scary and confusing.

The greatest and most simple mail is a card. Cards that say "Thinking about you" or "You are a special friend" or "Hello." There are countless stories of how people with Alzheimer's find these cards every day and read them as if it were the first time. Smile because this is a moment of joy anyone can give. Anyone can make a difference.

> *Society is always taken by surprise at any*
> *new example of common sense.*
> —Unknown

New-Found Treasure to Send

Walking, Walking, Walking

Walking does wonders! It is a great way to hit all five senses and relieve stress for you and the person with dementia. It is good exercise and helps us sleep better at night because of the vitamin D in the sun's rays.

When you walk, notice the simple things in nature, the peace and quiet. It also helps to put a few snacks in your pocket to share along the way. Walk at least once a day and work up to twice a day. I cannot emphasize enough the positive effects we all receive from walking. Even walking in the rain can be enjoyable for some.

> *At three o'clock every day Lindel would become very upset and want to get out of the facility. If we ignored his anger, it would just get worse and start affecting the other residents. We needed a solution, so I started a routine. At 1:30 every afternoon I would take Lindel and a few other people who were good walkers on a stroll through the neighborhood. Sometimes we would walk three times a day. The more we walked, the better the day went. If we didn't go for walks, Lindel would become extremely upset by 3:00 and want to go home. At this time, I would validate Lindel's feelings and say, "You know, I need a break from this place too. Can I join you?" He would rarely refuse because he knew he needed help finding his home. "Let me grab my coat*

and I will be right back" Then I would tell someone where I was going and to come look for us if we weren't back in an hour.

When we started our walk, I let him have an illusion of control by saying, "Which way should we go?" He usually chose the same direction every time, away from traffic and toward residential homes. While walking the first block, I would let him blow off some steam and make small talk. At the corner, I still gave him the illusion of control by saying again, "Now which way should we go?" I wouldn't hesitate with his decision, and more importantly, I showed him that I trusted him. Walking down the next block I would talk about his "treasures," which were fishing and his kids. "How many kids do you have?" "Boys or girls?" "Is it hard raising children?" "Can you give me any advice?" "Do you like to fish?" "You do? Well, I have tried it a few times and only caught the small ones. How do you catch the big ones?"

When we came to the next corner, I would say again, "Which way should we go?" and while he was deciding, I would innocently say, "I think this way looks good, what do you think?" (which gave him the illusion of choice). Because he didn't know which way to turn, he usually agreed with my suggestion. I started talking about different things, like the nature around us, a pretty house, the weather.

The main purpose was to get his mind off why he was so upset and get him to like and trust me. When we got to the next corner and were heading in the direction toward the facility, I would say, "You know what, I think I recognize something down this street. Let's go this way." On good days we walked right back to the facility. When he saw the facility, he would say, "Hey, that looks familiar!" Then we walked back inside the building and he would say, "This is the exact floor plan of my house. Thank you

*for bringing me home. What's your name again? It
was nice to meet you."*

*In my heart I was saying, "Yeah, you did it!"
On other days it would take more than four blocks,
and sometimes we would walk over a mile. I could
eventually get him back to the facility, but it wasn't
always easy.*

When we went on these walks, if someone walked too
far ahead, I didn't say, "Lindel, come back!" (especially
since he thinks the CIA is after him). I said, "Hey, wait up
for us!" (In other words, be a gentleman.)

Letting a person walk out the door when he wants to go
out can sometimes be a good thing. It not only gives an illusion of control but may be the only way to help him realize
that it is better inside. Then use the plan of action described
in the above story if he wants to keep on walking.

I don't recommend that just anyone should accompany
people with dementia on these walks. It takes a person who
is comfortable and confident with them and who can be
genuine with in tone of voice and body language. Be sure
the person knows the residents well.

Even though Lindel started as a problem resident, he
ended up being a blessing to others. We began the walking
program for him, but every resident benefited from it. It relieved stress and enabled other residents to walk, even in
the latest stages of the disease. Chair or bed alarms didn't
exist, because we didn't need them. We had very few in-
stances of falling because we walked, had an exercise routine every morning, and implemented a variety of physical
activities throughout the day (sweeping the back patio or
clearing the tables).

Relying on chair and bed alarms prevents a person from
retaining or building his muscles, so he is more likely to fall.
Because people with this disease think they are younger
than they actually are, they are more mobile than most
older people. Our group started out walking two blocks
and worked up to walking ten blocks a day. When you hear

about elderly ladies jumping over a fence without even tearing their skirt, now you know why—they are sixteen all over again!

> Q: *What did one flea say to the other flea?*
> A: *Should we walk or take a dog?*

New-Found Walking Routine

_____

_____

_____

_____

_____

_____

_____

_____

_____

_____

_____

_____

_____

_____

_____

_____

_____

_____

_____

_____

When In Doubt . . . Laugh

If your loved one fills the refrigerator with stuffed animals or hides fruit all over the house, laugh and continually remind yourself "So what!" Laughing enhances our sense of well-being, reduces stress, and improves our ability to survive a crisis. Physically, it increases circulation, reduces blood pressure, promotes brain functioning, relaxes muscles, reduces pain by increasing endorphins into the bloodstream, and stimulates the thymus gland, which improves the immune system.

I know this technical information isn't funny, like you perhaps thought this section would be, but hopefully it helps you understand the power of laughter. If you can't find anything to laugh about, just start laughing about nothing until you are laughing at yourself. If you laugh a lot, when you are older all your wrinkles will be in the right places!

If you haven't noticed, people with dementia can make incredibly witty and funny comments. I used to keep a small book in which I wrote down the funny things they did and said. This book was read by staff, and I feel it increased morale.

Another idea is to surround yourself with things that make you laugh: jokes, funny cards, comic strips, fun "stuff." Arrive at someone's bedside with a joke instead of complaining about your day. Whatever it takes to laugh, do it! You will be healthier for it, and so will the people around you, because laughing is contagious.

An activity person was having a discussion group with people who had dementia. One of the residents walked into the room and said loudly, "Oh, you think you're cute, but I know better. I saw you on the street downtown. You're a nasty hooker."

Obviously this could have been a very sticky situation, and everyone was wide-eyed waiting for a reaction. The activity person just started laughing, and soon everyone began to laugh. Eventually they forgot why they were laughing. The person could have been watching a TV show with hookers on it and felt hookers were in the building. The key is to understand that if we laugh more often, things could turn out differently.

The time to laugh is when we don't have time to laugh.
— Argus Poster

New-Found Funny

Share Your Life

When you have a few minutes, share your life. Even if the person cannot communicate, keep talking to her. Be sure the subject matter is positive and uplifting (getting married, new baby, weekend adventures). If you start talking about someone being sick, later in the day the person might worry about someone who she thinks is sick. Share your hobbies, pets, and children. People with dementia usually don't have the ability to go places and see people, because it can be very stressful. Think about it . . . when is the last time this person saw the moon and stars? Bring her the moon and the stars in a story.

> *I went to the ocean last week. We walked out on this jetty, which is a man-made surface of huge stones going out about a mile into the ocean. The wind blew so hard, you should have seen our wild hair when we got back to our cars. We couldn't even get our fingers through it. The waves were huge, and they crashed against the rocks with such force that if you were close to the edge you got soaked. The water tasted salty, too. It was like eating salt straight out of the container.*
>
> *We went all the way to the end of this jetty and looked at the endless horizon of water. Ice-blue water, just like in the movies. Every once in a while you could see fishing boats and then they would be*

*gone behind the enormous waves. Then we took our
shoes off and walked along the beach. The water was
so cold it numbed my feet, and it actually hurt. We
picked up broken shells, and I even saw a deep red
starfish on one of the larger rocks.*

*We ate at a near-by restaurant. They had the
best clam chowder with these big onion rings. What
else did we do? . . . Oh yeah, we took a walk along
the beach that night. When I closed my eyes, it was
almost scary, because the noise of the waves was so
loud I felt like they were going to crash on me. I
must tell you it was an amazing experience.*

Have you been to the ocean before?"

*When I had my first child, I was working in an Alz-
heimer's facility. Within a week after my daughter
was born, I brought her in and let the residents hold
her. A staff member asked, "Aren't you afraid they
might drop her?" I said reassuringly, "They know
exactly what they are holding. It will be OK." Even
a lady in the latest stage of Alzheimer's held her and
perked up a bit, making baby noises, and clearly said
"beautiful baby." A moment I will never forget.*

*If you wouldn't feel comfortable letting others
hold your baby, just sit beside them with the baby in
your arms. They love to just touch the baby's little
fingers. When my little girl got older, I brought her
in and put her in the middle of the room and let her
play for all to see. The residents gave me a gift with
their smiling faces. Even today my daughter enjoys
going to care facilities and singing for the people.*

*My mission is to tell others how we take too
many things away from those with dementia to be
on the safe side. We have literally taken away the
most precious gifts we can give.*

If you play an instrument, crochet, have a litter of pup-
pies, tell a good story, or make great chocolate chip cookies,

share these talents and irresistible things with people in facilities. Watching you do something you're good at may be a priceless gift to someone.

Another wonderful idea is to videotape your babies or children and bring it to the facility for the people to watch. Make sure you don't come in large numbers, like a big band or a full choir. Too much stimulation or noise causes stress and confusion. Small groups are better, and giving time one-on-one is best. We all have talents, and I know where you can find an appreciative audience.

Discover the magic within yourself!

New-Found Shared Treasure from Your Life

_____

_____

_____

_____

_____

_____

_____

_____

_____

_____

_____

_____

_____

_____

_____

_____

Drink Up!

We need to make an effort to keep people with Alzheimer's hydrated. They lose their sense of thirst or are unable to tell you they are thirsty, so we need to remind them to drink water. Just setting a glass of water in front of them isn't enough. Give them a reason to drink or cue them to drink. "Wow, it sure is hot today." "It will feel so good to wet your whistle."

If this doesn't work, place your hand over the other person's hand and assist him to drink the water. If someone is dehydrated or malnutritioned, he will function at a lower level. Possibly he will display behaviors similiar to those associated with Alzheimer's disease but not actually have the disease at all.

So drink up!

Luey: Sam, you know the worst thing about growing old?
Sam: No . . . What's that?
Luey: What's what?

Joys are our wings.

New-Found Desired Beverage

_____

_____

_____

_____

_____

_____

_____

_____

_____

_____

_____

_____

_____

_____

_____

_____

_____

_____

_____

_____

_____

_____

_____

_____

_____

_____

Saturating Obsessions

When a person has Alzheimer's, she might start obsessing about various things (washing her hair, hoarding dishes, peeling potatoes). If she is at the dinner table and constantly taking other people's cups or plates, just give her extra cups and plates when serving her. It doesn't feel normal to us to hoard items, but who cares as long as the person gets what she desires in the end? Feel free to indulge, and even, saturate, her obsessions.

> *Dowell was obsessed with shoelaces. He would take them out of other people's shoes and tie them in knots. First we tried taking away all the shoelaces and distracting him with activities or changing the subject. It didn't work. Then we gave him a box full of shoelaces and some shoes so he could do as he pleased. Not only was he busy for hours, but he was content.*

> *Alice frequently commented how she would like to peel potatoes. At first everyone was concerned she would cut herself with the knife. When they found out peeling potatoes was a habit of a lifetime for Alice, they decided to bring her a five-gallon pail full of potatoes, and she peeled until she could peel no more.*

Simplify, simplify, simplify. If you're concerned about Alice's safety, you could boil the potatoes first and have her scrape the skin off with a table knife (she might complain it isn't sharp enough or this isn't the right way to peel potatoes). Just bringing her the potatoes might be enough. Keep in mind that you need to know the person well and what her abilities are, but please give her a chance to fulfill her wishes, which is what you would want.

When faced with a mountain, I will not quit!
I will keep on striving until I climb over,
find a pass through, tunnel underneath,
or simply stay and turn the mountain into a gold mine–
with God's help!

New-Found Obsession and Solution

_____
_____
_____
_____
_____
_____
_____
_____
_____
_____
_____
_____
_____
_____
_____
_____
_____

Spreading Holidays throughout the Year

Holidays are usually very stressful for everyone, especially for those with dementia. Not only do we take them out of their familiar environment but we also invite everyone over and ask them to be normal once again with the whole family. Indeed, holidays are usually the time when families first see that something is wrong.

Please change this stressful pattern. Spread the holidays throughout the whole year. On Sunday go to the Christmas church service. The next week invite one family for dinner. The next month open presents one night, and then once or twice a month, schedule one family to visit and open presents. If your loved one lives in a facility, the same applies. Keep events simple, with a few people in a familiar environment, and enjoy the simple blessings.

When a person with Alzheimer's disease is still living at home, I encourage you to rethink the holiday tradition so it can be more enjoyable for him or her, less stressful for the care provider, and easier for the family.

Steps to Help Get through the Holidays

1. Call a family meeting before the holidays. Discuss traditions that *must* be continued and traditions that the family would be willing to change.

2. Make a *must-do* list and a *should-do* list. For example, I *must* buy gifts for my children. I *should* bake some holiday treats, but I *could* buy them at a local bakery. Try to do only those items that are on your must-do list.

3. If large gatherings are uncomfortable for your loved one with Alzheimer's disease, but the family must all be together, set up a schedule for the day. Assign each family member an hour to be with your loved one, to take him outside for a walk if he is restless, to take him into the bedroom for much-needed quiet time. Make sure he is never left "alone in a crowd." The day will be much easier if someone is next to him saying things like "Here comes your son, Joe, and his daughter, Megan." "Dinner is on the table. I will walk you to the dining room." "Mom is taking the ham out of the oven. She will be here in just a minute."

4. Ask for help. This sounds much easier than it is, especially if you are the kind of person who is determined to do it all yourself. Try asking for small things at first. Maybe you *must* cook the turkey and the family's favorite stuffing, and you *should* make the trimmings, but you *could* ask each guest to help by bringing a vegetable or dessert.

5. Put yourself first. Treat yourself during the holidays. Take your loved one to an adult daycare an extra day each week. Take your neighbor up on the offer to take her out for drive. Take a nap. Read a good book. Exercise. Take deep breaths. Take a walk in the woods.

6. It is important for family and friends to understand your situation and have realistic expectations. You might choose to write a letter:

Dear Family and Friends,

As you are aware, Joe was diagnosed with Alzheimer's disease —— years ago. We are looking forward to seeing you this holiday season, and we thought it might help for you to understand our situation before you arrive.

I am enclosing a picture of Joe. As you can see, he has changed quite a bit since you last saw him. Not only has he changed in looks, but some other things you might notice are —— (fill in the blank; for example, he does not know the people close to him, walks aimlessly in a circle through the living room, dining room, and kitchen). I hope you understand that he may not recognize you. Please don't be offended. I hope you will treat Joe as you normally do. A smile and a hug mean so much. We cherish your friendship and are eager to see you.

7. Your local Alzheimer's Association chapter has many wonderful ideas for gifts for a person with Alzheimer's disease. Look in the telephone book for the chapter nearest you.

Families need to work together to survive this disease. I've heard many stories about how the oldest sibling is responsible for the parent, or the daughter and daughter in-laws take on the responsibility. This journey cannot be taken alone. Each sibling needs to play a role in taking care of a parent. Maybe the son handles the finances, and the daughter sets up a schedule for when different families and friends visit or take care of person.

One family that I worked with put together a calendar with a person's picture above the month. The person in the picture was responsible for care that month. Maybe it would work better for you to go by weeks. The point is that no one person can do this alone. Only by working together can we become strong.

*If, as Herod, we fill our lives with the things, and again with
things; if we consider ourselves so unimportant that we must fill
every moment of our lives with action, when will we have the
time to make the long, slow journey across the desert as did the
Magi? Or sit and watch the stars as did the shepherds? Or
brood over the coming of the child as did Mary? For each one of
us, there is a desert to travel. A star to discover. And a being
within ourselves to bring to life.*

—Unknown

New-Found Holiday Tradition

Keys to Visiting

Relax and enjoy your visit. If you are having a good time, the person with Alzheimer's will too. Please don't stop visiting because the person no longer recognizes you or is unable to talk back. Your presence does make a difference.

Pointers

- Begin each visit by introducing yourself and addressing your loved one by name. It's hard not to be offended if she doesn't recognize or remember your name. But realize it's part of the disease process, and with support, understanding, and encouragement you are more likely to enjoy the time you have together.

- If you are visiting in a facility, acknowledge other residents as if they were close friends. If you accept the other people in the facility, the person with Alzheimer's may adjust better to living there. Better yet, take a few minutes to share the fond memories you have about your loved one with staff and other residents.

- Don't rush your family member. Allow him enough time to respond to questions or directions.

- Consider the person's interest and abilities,

and even discuss, if possible, what he would enjoy doing. For example, if he expresses interest in gardening, offer to take him to a flower garden or give him flowers regularly. In the later stages of the disease, you could bring a plant, but you should realize that you have to be the one who will water and take care of it. The staff and other residents will enjoy it too.

• Plan activities ahead of time, then be flexible according to the person's mood or ability level during the visit. When planning an outing, be sure to keep it simple with little stimulation. Maybe it's just going for a drive in the country, walking in a park, or having a picnic in a quiet area. The fewer people involved and the simpler the tasks, the more enjoyment you will both have.

• Do simple familiar activities, such as going for walks, looking at photo albums, snacking on favorite treats, or just enjoying each other's company.

• If your loved one becomes anxious or upset, remain calm and assist him to a quiet place, away from stimulating areas like the dining room or activity room. Even before you begin visiting, find a quiet, calm place to sit.

• Avoid conversations dealing with the "here and now." Something like "Anna told me she visited with you yesterday" relies on short-term memory. Use your family member's long-term memory instead: "Anna, your sister, is a pretty neat lady. She called me yesterday and we talked about . . ." In your conversations always include the relationship of the person after the name, because your family member may remember he has a sister but cannot remember his sister's name.

• "Live their truth."

- Visit in small groups; actually one-on-one is the best.

- Visit as a third person. Instead of saying "Mom," say her name. She thinks her kids are little, and now you might be lying because you can't be her kid. You're too old! She remembers you, but she remembers you when you were little.

People will forget what you said,
People will forget what you did,
but they will never forget
how you made them feel.

New-Found Treasure while Visiting

Saying Good-Bye

If you want to leave for a short time, give your loved one a reason for your departure. "I need to use the restroom" is a great reason. You can use this excuse even if don't need to use the restroom. Or you can say, "I need to run an errand. I will be back in a little while." If she needs more detail, don't be afraid to say you will be back in ten minutes and leave for twenty minutes. Since her sense of time is affected by Alzheimer's, this response works.

If you don't give her a reason, she might be looking for you and become uneasy during the short time you are gone. Remember to use a genuine tone of voice and an easygoing manner. If you're comfortable with saying good-bye, she is more likely to be comfortable with it. Reassure her and be vague: "I'll be back soon." Choose a place where she wouldn't want to go: "I have to go to the dentist."

Possible Ways to Say Good-Bye

- Husband-and-wife scenario: "John, I've really enjoyed our visit, but I have a hair appointment soon. You're going to have lunch here, so enjoy. I'll see you later. I love you." Your answer will vary. Just remember to talk in a reassuring tone and give a reason for your departure that your spouse will believe.

- Parent or sibling scenario: "I'm glad we had this time together. Take care and I'll see you soon. I love you."

- Friend-to-friend scenario: "Francis, it is so good to see you again. We should do this more often. I need to run some errands, but thanks for a wonderful afternoon. I'll visit you again soon, Francis." When leaving, it helps to give hugs, a reassuring touch, or familiar words that say you care.

- Staff scenario: Excuse yourself by saying, "Lunch is going to be ready in about fifteen minutes. Why not relax until then? Would you like some music while you wait?" Give residents time to respond, and respect their wishes. If you have two different requests, you make the decision and tell the other person that next time the music will be off, or whatever is appropriate for your situation. Then reassure them that someone will come get them when lunch is ready.

At work, you think of the children you have left at home. At home, you think of the work you've left unfinished. Such a struggle is unleashed within yourself. Your heart is rent.

—Golda Meir

New-Found Way to Say Good-Bye

_____

_____

_____

_____

_____

_____

_____

_____

Outings with Less Stress

Simplify outings by just going on short country drives, visiting friends at their house, watching children play at a park, feeding ducks, or going for a walk in a quiet neighborhood. Avoid eating out at restaurants, especially during prime hours. If you really want to go out to eat, ask for a private room away from the noise and rush. Avoid malls and zoos; these places just aren't familiar and have too much stimulation.

On the other hand, if a person with dementia is clearly enjoying herself at a mall, then you know it is OK. Use the rule of thumb: If it works, it works! If it doesn't, it doesn't! To figure out whether it works or not, be aware of the person's emotions. If she seems really confused or anxious, you know you will have to change and try something else or simplify your outing.

If she lives in a facility, call and ask the staff how she is doing when you get home. Try anything once and don't assume she won't like something. This way you won't miss out on a possible moment of joy.

> Gladys had to leave her farmhouse and move into a nearby facility. She had always been a very proper, well-mannered lady. The family decided to take her out for a drive.
>
> When they brought her back to the facility, she would not go inside. She wanted to go home. The

staff insisted this was her home, and she needed to get inside. After a while they resorted to forcing her back into the facility, but that didn't work either. Even though she was a little lady with gray hair, weighing only 100 pounds, she won that battle.

A third person came along and observed the situation and nonchalantly walked up to the lady and said, "Gladys, your daughters are inside waiting to eat lunch with you. Are you hungry?" She said yes and walked inside the building. As easy as that.

Unfortunately the family is scared to take their mother on an outing again because of this incident. This happens all too often, and we keep taking things away because we are scared of what might happen. Soon the person with dementia ends up with very little in her life. In this situation, we should treasure the solution that was found and use it over and over again.

A group of people just got back from a bus trip, and one gentleman wouldn't get off the bus. Many people tried to coax him off the bus, but after an hour he still sat there. A staff person remembered that he didn't like loud music. They turned up the radio, and he immediately got off the bus. Goes to show, we need to be creative all over again!

Celebrate the Seasons

If your loved one is unable to go on outings, celebrate the seasons inside. For example, in the spring bring in baby animals, plant a flowering bush outside his window, talk about the farmers in the fields, or bring in a pot of tulips so he can enjoy the miracle of growth. In the summer, bring him fresh strawberries, open a window to give the free gift of fresh warm air, sit in the backyard, soak his feet in a wading pool while drinking a glass of fresh lemonade, or stop and smell the roses or the lilac bushes. In the fall, share the harvest, the turning leaves, or take a nature walk. In the winter, break off icicles, just like you did when you were little, and share the experience. Together talk about the feeling of the cold, wet icicle melting in your mouth and slipping through your fingers. Stop and see the miracles in the simple things of daily living. I bet you will receive as many gifts of joy as you give away.

Why do mother kangaroos hate rainy days?
Because their kids have to play inside.

New-Found Outing That Brings Joy

_____

_____

_____

_____

_____

_____

_____

_____

_____

_____

_____

_____

_____

_____

_____

_____

_____

_____

Face the Challenges

There are a variety of challenges you will have to face head on. I encourage you to take everyday situations more lightly and choose your battles.

Loss of Emotional Control

Along with short-term memory loss, a person with Alzheimer's loses the ability to control his emotions. This is why you hear stories about the sweetest, most-pleasant people having emotional outbursts (tearful, terrified, frustrated, angry, depressed, suspicious).

When someone is very upset about something, stay calm and say what he wants to hear. In other words, tell him he is right, and you will help him the best that you can. It is always easier to prevent someone from becoming really upset rather than dealing with the situation after he is upset. If you witness a gentleman who is upset or two men fighting, walk up to them and extend your hand for a handshake and ask if there is anything you can do to help. A handshake is a friendly gesture that brings down the wall, and men respond very well to it.

Wandering

Wandering is another aspect of this disease, and it can usually be explained because in their minds those with dementia are constantly trying to make sense of their environment, wanting to find something that is familiar, or they may be anxious. There are many reasons why they wander, and I encourage you not to choose this as one of your battles because it is so common to this disease. Instead you might modify the environment to make wandering safe.

Hitting

Hitting is something else that occurs with dementia sufferers, and I feel it is directly related to our not understanding their needs and adding too much stress to their lives. Sometimes the only way for them to communicate is to hit. If they hit, they could be saying "stop putting pressures on me and change the way you do things." Some caregivers who work with people who have dementia on a daily basis have never been hit. When I was working on the floor eight hours a day, I was never hit. They understood and responded to the power of a genuine touch, tone of voice, and understanding. Much of what they do is a reaction from outside stimulation.

Losing Items

When a person with dementia forgets where he puts things, he automatically thinks someone must have taken the items, so his next thought is that he needs to hide his things. Because of short-term memory loss, he forgets where he hid the items. It becomes a vicious never-ending cycle. One health-care provider told about some of the strange places she found things: an iron in the oven, ice cream in the linen closet, a watch in the sugar bowl, milk in the freezer, jewelry in the microwave, and underwear in a purse. Some of these hiding places make sense if you think about where the person might be living in his mind. Accept the fact that many things will get misplaced, so have six of everything for backup!

> *In a facility, they started losing very expensive items like glasses, dentures, and hearing aids. Families became very upset, and staff spent countless hours try-*

ing to find these items. One day they walked unex-
pectedly into a gentleman's room while he was trying
to hide these items. Guess where his hiding place was.

You couldn't begin to guess because he hid these
items in the ceiling. Yes, he figured out that the tiles
in the ceiling could be moved. He stepped on a chair
and tucked them neatly out of sight.

So my recommendation to you is to stop trying to find things. Items that are lost usually show up sooner or later, and in this case the staff could have looked forever, wasting much valuable time. Instead get a marker board and write "LOST" at the top of it. When anyone is trying to find something, write it down.

> *There are some things you learn best in calm,*
> *and some in storm.*
>
> —Willa Cather

Fragmented Sleeping

Whether they have dementia or not, as people get older, their sleeping patterns change. They might go to bed at 8:00, get up at 1:00, stay up for a couple of hours, go back to sleep until 6:00, and then take two naps during the day.

Fragmented sleeping is an issue that evolves with age. Fatigue is a major cause of the many challenges we face. In the past we have resorted to keeping people up all day, thinking they will sleep better at night, but the functioning ability is greatly lowered during the day because of fatigue. I cannot stress enough how important it is for people to take at least one nap a day.

> *Right after lunch staff encouraged residents to be ac-*
> *tive for about a half an hour to improve metabolism.*
> *Then around 1:00 every afternoon I would read a*
> *short story about a positive event (weddings, love,*
> *children, old-time memories). I would read slowly*
> *and in a monotone voice. If eighteen out of the*

twenty residents were sleeping, I did my job well! A quick cat nap will improve the rest of the day.

Allow the person to sleep in mornings. If I lived in a facility and someone woke me up before 7:30, I would be agitated and disoriented too. Some of us are morning people, and some of us are night owls. We are made from different molds.

Suggestions to Help People Get Their Z's

- Expose them to sunlight—there is vitamin D in the sun rays to help us sleep better.

- Keep people physically active during the day.

- Establish a calming evening routine.

- With a little research you can find foods to eat that help us sleep better at night.

- Eliminate stimulating activities after 7:00 P.M.

- Put on an extra blanket an hour after the person has fallen asleep to keep him warm. Being cold is one reason why people don't sleep well. Remember, this disease makes people colder than cold.

- If person is used to sleeping with someone else, get a body pillow and spray it with the scent of the other person.

- Read poetry or rhymes or sing quiet songs as an evening activity. A steady beat or rhythm is like a lullaby at night.

- Use a white noise machine; its subtle noise is soothing to fall asleep to.

- Fulfill habits of a lifetime, such as sleeping with a feather pillow, sleeping with the fan on, sleeping in a pitch-dark room or with a night-light.

- If possible, allow a person to sleep in his own bed, not a hospital bed.

- A common reason why people wake up in the middle of the night is to use the bathroom, but a person with Alzheimer's might be unable to tell you that, so it should be the first thing you ask.

- Let the person wake up on his own in the morning.

- Walking, walking, walking!

If the spouse is the care provider, giving medication to the person with dementia may help both of them get much-needed sleep. You may want to consult with your family doctor about this issue.

> *"That we are not much sicker and much madder than we are*
> *is due exclusively to that most blessed and*
> *blessing of all natural graces, sleep."*
> —Aldous Huxley

Sexuality

Sexuality, or intimacy, is often ignored. However, intimacy and being sexually active are a very normal part of adult life. Control of sexuality is thought to be located in the limbic system, which is damaged with Alzheimer's disease, so the person may be sexually active or may lose interest in sex. Intimacy should not be confused with sex. Many times a person simply craves the touch of another person. Those who need touch the most receive touch less often. Staff must be trained to touch appropriately and frequently, including holding hands or simply touching their faces or patting their backs.

Understanding Life Habits

> *Does this person have an affectionate family?*
>
> *Has the person ever slept in bed alone?*

What is the person's sexual orientation?

Is there any history of sexual abuse?

At-home caregivers may struggle with the changing needs of a person with Alzheimer's disease. The spouse may choose to sleep in a separate bed or bedroom so she can get enough sleep. Mary, a woman in her early sixties who is caring for her husband, told this story:

> *George and I had a wonderful day. He was more alert than normal. We visited our daughter and had a picnic by the lake. On the ride home, George was able to respond to my comments and seemed very happy and relaxed. Once home, we went into the bedroom to get ready for bed. As I started to undress, George started crying and pushing me out the door. After calming him down, it became apparent that he was confused—he believed I was our daughter. The fact that he thought our daughter was undressing in front of him and that he didn't recognize me as his wife was the most devastating thing that has happened so far in this disease. I had hoped that this might have been be a night when I could once again sleep in his arms. I ended up in the guest room, alone." Mary is rightfully grieving for the husband she is losing.*

> *Bob, who has Alzheimer's, and Betty, his wife, went to a restaurant with several other family members one evening. Bob and Betty were seated next to each other. Suddenly Bob felt lost and could not see Betty. Betty simply turned to him and said, "I am right here, Bob. I'm Betty, your wife." Bob, with much love and adoration in his eyes, touched Betty's face lightly and commented, "And you're so beautiful." What a blessing for Betty to know that Bob thought she was beautiful after fifty-nine years of marriage!*

Although the sexual part of the marriage may be over, with education and support, the long-shared intimacy between two people may be sustained. Be sure both parties are capable of consensual sex.

Every situation is different, and know that you are not alone. Sharing your story in a support group and with others will help. No one can get through these loses alone.

The best and most beautiful things in the world cannot be seen or touched but are felt in the heart.

—Helen Keller

Pain

Pain can often be a culprit for such behavioral symptoms as generalized irritability, pacing, increased wandering, anxiety, resistance to care activities, and depressive-like symptoms. The person suffering from dementia may not be able to verbally articulate successfully that she is feeling pain. It may be difficult for her to differentiate pain from another stimulus. She does know, however that she is feeling discomfort.

As caregivers, we must often make assumptions about the individual with dementia. We do this with observational information about the person and comparing it to other experiences we have had. This is an important tool but cannot be the only tool. Pain can be assessed by using simple questioning and screening tools. Many can use a pain intensity scale. Caregivers may want to try out several versions. Some caregivers find it helpful to use an intensity scale with faces, similar to what children are offered in hospitals. Sometimes we need to find the right words (those that make sense to the individual with dementia) to use in order to describe the pain. Asking the person whether she "hurts" or "feels badly" in an area of her body may be more helpful, or talking with family members and asking how she has historically acted when in pain.

In addition, it is helpful to review a person's medical history to determine whether there are current or past medical problems that may in fact cause her to be in pain now. Arthritis, osteoporosis, chronic back pain, gout, stroke, history of multiple fractures, or diabetes are examples of conditions that can cause both acute and chronic pain. These need to be reviewed with the individual's health-care provider, so that the appropriate interventions are pursued.

At times, it is so difficult to differentiate pain as a source of agitation for an individual versus another source that a caregiver may need to discuss a trial of regularly scheduled pain medication with the health-care provider. Monitoring the use of regularly scheduled pain medication and assessing an decrease in suspected pain-related behaviors is helpful in determining whether pain is present and then relieved, or whether there may in fact be another source of agitation.

Most individuals with dementia also respond to non-medication type remedies. These include hot and cold treatments, relaxation, distraction, and massage. They should be explored in conjunction with pain medication with the individual's health care provider.

If their behavior is different today than yesterday,
it is probably not the disease but pain!

New-Found Challenges and How You Faced Them

_____

_____

_____

_____

_____

_____

_____

_____

Letting Go of Expectations

In the middle stages of Alzheimer's, a person's developmental level is eight years old. As the disease progresses, their developmental level is five years old and younger. In the late stages of Alzheimer's, it is three years of age and younger. If you have grandchildren or children three years old or younger, watch what they are able to do, and a person with Alzheimer's can probably do it too. In the very final stages of this disease, she will do what a baby starts out doing. The first thing a baby can do is hold his head up and the next is to smile. These are the last things a person with Alzheimer's can do. As the disease progresses, her development regresses in almost the same way as an infant's grows.

The same seems to apply for inhibitions; where a child has not yet formed inhibitions, the adult with dementia loses her inhibitions. For example, my one-year-old daughter pours milk over her food and plays in it. She wants me to sing the same song over and over again. Up to the age of two years old, both my children frequently got out of bed after I put them to bed and woke up often in the middle of the night.

This awareness of the challenges that occur in each developmental level, helps me understand a person with Alzheimer's. There is definitely a difference, though, in the language and tone of voice (high pitch) we use for babies compared to the language and tone of voice (low pitch) we use for older people. This also does not mean we treat older people like children. This means we understand and accept the capabilities of a person with Alzheimer's.

> *A staff person explained how difficult it was to have people with Alzheimer's living in the same area as people who are cognitively well but physically ill. She said it made a huge difference when they opened up a Alzheimer's special care unit. Before, residents would yell when a person with dementia came into their room. Now in this new unit she was seeing three people in the same room not aware of each other's presence. One person was rummaging through the closet, another person was tearing up Kleenex, and the third person was sitting on the bed picking at the bed spread. She compared it to a preschool setting because everyone was very content doing his own thing in the same room. There is less stress for a person when he is in an environment with other people acting the same way as he does. Alzheimer's facilities are a good thing.*

A person with dementia needs structure and routine, as children do. When a child is out of her everyday environment and routine, she will either run wild or cling to you. If she misses her nap, she is cranky. There is a theory that a person with dementia has difficulty learning new things. The solution is structure, routine, and repetition. Doing the same thing at the same time of day makes it easier for the person to adapt to something new. Having knowledge about the person's habits of a lifetime and having a routine every day is the key if you want less stress and more success.

> *Cecelia lived in a retirement facility, and was usually well oriented. She walked to the dining room for all her meals. This facility had assigned seats for everyone, but on this particular day visitors sat at her table. When she got up to leave, she commented on how lovely the company was in this restaurant, and*

then she wanted to know how she was going to get home. Just changing the people sitting across from her changed her whole environment and caused confusion.

*And there are those who give and
know not pain in giving, nor do they seek joy,
nor give with mindfulness of virtue; They give as a Yonder
Valley the myrtle breathes it's fragrance into space. Through
the hands of such as these God speaks, and from behind their
eyes He smiles upon the earth.*

— Kahlil Gibran

New-Found Structure and Routine

_____
_____
_____
_____
_____
_____
_____
_____
_____
_____
_____
_____
_____
_____
_____
_____
_____

Spiritual Well-Being

Religion could be an important part of a person's life. How can we enrich his life through religion? As an example, it's not just being Lutheran, but it's knowing his personal rituals to uphold his beliefs. Reading a devotion before going to bed may be a habit of a lifetime for him. Saying prayer before mealtimes may kick start him that it is time to eat. Reading certain Scriptures that he has heard over and over will evoke memories and offer comfort. Displaying significant spiritual symbols in his environment (angels, cross, Mary, Last Supper) may fill a void. Seeing a picture of Jesus when he opens his eyes, may bring comfort.

It's wonderful how many hymns seem to be universal for different religions, like "Amazing Grace" and "How Great Thou Art." Older people know many hymns by heart and singing these hymns offers comfort to those with dementia. Even though they may not be able to attend church, some aspects of church may be brought to them. For example, in the Catholic Church people are designated to bring communion to those who cannot attend church. Communion is such a strong symbol within the Catholic faith and by itself may evoke memories of spirituality. Search a person's history. Figure out how you can fulfill his spiritual needs.

> *Reverend Joseph was a kind gentleman with Alz-*
> *heimer's disease. When you would talk with him, he*
> *would lose his words and have difficulty communi-*
> *cating his thoughts. What was wonderful, however,*
> *was that at the end of every activity he was com-*
> *pelled to close with a prayer. When he was praying,*
> *words would spill out with such feeling and elo-*
> *quence that we were moved from each experience. It*
> *was a blessing to have him with us.*

Ron Kitterman is the chaplain of a large care facility. He expresses so eloquently what spiritual well-being means to the person with Alzheimer's and how God fits into the picture. His information has become the glue that holds my words together and I would like to summarize and share these thoughts with you.

Spiritual Well-Being

How we understand and value "spirituality" affects the way we cope with the challenges involved with dementia. A healthy spirituality will ease the struggles that you and the person with dementia face, but spirituality is not about faith reversing or curing the disease process. Arthur Freeman suggests that "[Spiritual] Well-being to some extent has to do with being well, but it has more to do with existing well in the midst of whatever life brings to one. Thus there can be well-being in the midst of suffering."

Spiritual well-being is not the same as being well. Spiritual well-being is finding meaning in what life presents to us, finding that meaning brings about healing. The next step is to constantly ask yourself, "What does this person need to enjoy life at the fullest, right now, given the state of his health?" We can still care for a body that has spirit and that is capable of well-being even if it is not capable of being well.

Healing should not be confused with finding a cure. Healing begins with our acceptance of dementia and the changes it brings and by facing the disease head on. Healing comes in many different forms. In the midst of suffering, a loving God longs to meet our deepest needs of our heart. God will give us meaning and a sense of well-being in whatever comes our way. When we aspire and strive to walk through the pain, peace will truly deepen, and as we receive God's grace, we will go to the core of our spiritual journey.

How do we come to terms with what it means to have spiritual well-being in our own lives? Our journey can become easier as we discover what it means to have a sense of well-being. When we face our deepest longings, difficult feelings, questions, fears, confusion, and pain with dementia and in our own life, this will lead to our awareness of what it means to deepen our spiritual journey. Where does God fit into the world of dementia? In a book called *God Never Forgets*, Don McKim writes, "God sees the suffering from the inside; God does not look at it from the outside, as through a window. God is internally related to the suffering of the people. God enters fully into the hurtful situation and makes it (God's) own."

Our culture tells us our value is based on what we do, and therefore our worth is based on external, not internal, things. Regardless of how our culture and others try to dictate to us how to live, we need to try and come to terms with how God sees us. Even though society tells us that if we lose autonomy we are no longer human, I feel that our value is based in and from God. We are like aluminum pop cans. We start out worth a nickel, and when we are done holding the contents, we are still worth a nickel. If we believe we are made in the image of God, then we are truly a reflection of God. Our spirituality absolutely affects us. It is the very essence of our faith. Faith is seeing light with the eyes of our heart when the eyes of our body see only darkness ahead.

God will remember
even if the person with dementia forgets
and the caregiver falls exhausted!
—Ron Kitterman

Walk by faith, not by sight.
—II Corinthians 5:7

New-Found Offering of Spiritual Well-Being

Find the Blessings

It's understandable that the children of someone with Alzheimer's want their mom back. We want our parents to remember who we are. We go to great lengths to try to restart the part of the brain that has truly died. We stand with our mom in front of a mirror and say, "Mom, don't you see that I look a lot like you? I am your daughter, Viola." The reply usually goes like this: "You're not my daughter. You are an old lady." If you look deeper into this reply, you realize that she does remember she has children, but her children are young. Remember, people with Alzheimer's have lost the last twenty to fifty years of their lives.

If we continue to insist that we are her children, a wall may go up, and the parent may be thinking, "Who is this impostor in my room?" Again, we have to be the ones to change, which may mean visiting as a third person. Instead of saying "mom," start out with, "Alice, it's Viola, and I stopped by to see you." Then maybe these next stories can become your own.

> *The mother has Alzheimer's. She has a daughter whom she has been fighting with for the last twenty years. The daughter only has hurt feelings and carries much anger toward her mother. When the daughter learned more about the disease, she realized her mom had probably lost fifty years. The daughter introduced herself by saying, "Hi, Marga-*

ret, my name is Judy, and I found your photo album. I was hoping you could tell me about the little blond girl in this picture." The mother told the daughter stories about herself she had never heard before. Stories that were filled with love and adoration for this wonderful little girl. The daughter was again reminded of her mother's love and given precious memories to hold that replaced the memories and the anger from the last twenty years. When this woman loses the ability to talk, her daughter can give back the memories she has been given. This was truly a blessing.

Jean's dad, Harold, was always at work when she was growing up. Harold had little time for his family. He tended to drink and was physically abusive on occasion when his children were young. Now Harold has Alzheimer's disease and lives in a care facility. When Jean visits, Harold does not recognize her, nor does he give any indication he knows she is a familiar person to him.

However, the staff tells Jean that her father frequently asks if Jean is coming to visit, and when he is displeased, he calls out for Jean to help him. One afternoon, Jean found him staring out the window with a very sad look on his face. "Hi, Dad. What's wrong?" Jean asked. Harold told her about his little girl, his daughter, and how much he missed her. "I don't think she loves me," Harold said. Jean asked Harold to tell her more about his daughter. What she heard was a tale about a father who did love his daughter but didn't know how to show it. Harold said, "I just wish I could tell her how much I love her." With tears in her eyes, Jean said, "She knows, Dad, she knows." The blessing for Jean was discovering that her dad did love her. He just never knew how to show it.

Some parents may have difficulty showing their love to their own children. It's easier to brag about their children to other people. Grasp the moment and search for the blessings in every situation. You will be surprised at what you find.

> *Sally always wanted to go home. She thought she was just staying at this facility for a little while until she felt better. Even though she had been living in this facility for two years, she thought she had been there for just a couple of weeks. There is a blessing here.*

You have a very important role to help a person with dementia to continue to live with a smile and give back treasured memories even when she loses the ability to communicate. You need to try to accept the negative and look for the blessings, as simple as they are. Once you do this, you will find you have more energy to make the changes to enjoy the moments.

> *The best advice for stress is this:*
> *you may not be able to avoid suffering,*
> *but you don't have to wallow in it. Pain comes into everybody's*
> *life, but misery is optional.*
> *Stress may be a given factor, but your attitude can change the*
> *way it affects you.*
>
> — Barbara Johnson

New-Found Blessing

_____

_____

_____

_____

_____

_____

Taking Care of Yourself

I thought about placing this section at the beginning of the book *and* at the end to emphasize that you need to take care of yourself before you can take care of someone else. No matter what your situation, start now and get involved with your own life once again. Take time to do the things you love to do, be with people who make you feel good, and pamper—or better yet, spoil—yourself often. Just as we need to relieve stress for a person with dementia, you need to find ways to relieve stress in your own life.

It is proven that stress adversely affects brain functioning. You know you have stress when you find the cereal box in the refrigerator and the milk in the cupboard. Admit it, we have all done that once in a while. Reducing stress helps us function better.

Even when you don't feel like it, smile, because just smiling lifts your spirit and relieves stress. Exercising is a great way to relieve stress and increases blood flow to the brain. Meditating twenty minutes in the morning and at night will help you relax. One way of meditating is a "centering prayer," a positive strengthening word that you repeat slowly until you are resting with that word. Do activities that you enjoy to stimulate your brain in a healthy way.

Too much stimulation to the brain will cause stress, and not enough stimulation causes boredom or depression. It is important to find a balance. Another word for it is to get into a "flow state," which means you are active yet relaxed in your activity. Also have two to three activities you like, so you are challenging your brain in different areas.

Of course, eat good foods, lower your fat intake, and drink lots of water (six cups a day). Get lots of rest! If your loved one is having fragmented sleeping patterns and waking up in the middle of the night for a couple of hours, you need to sleep when he sleeps. This might mean napping at 10:00 in the morning.

Most importantly, take time off from caregiving—at least two days a week. I hear many reasons why people feel like they can't take time off. The fact is that if you don't take care of yourself first, you will soon be less healthy than the person with dementia.

We say that the person with Alzheimer's is the victim, but really the one taking care of the person with Alzheimer's is the victim. It is not unusual for the spouse to die before the person with dementia. When someone is diagnosed with Alzheimer's, the family should become patients too. Alzheimer's disease is understandably devastating to families. It creates tension and stress for even the most solid families. It's overwhelming when you are suddenly responsible for finances, the house, and for a person who is dependent on you for the most basic needs (eating, grooming, bathing, dressing). Many times, the best solution is to find a good care facility. Seek help from others so you are able take care of yourself!

Helping Hands

The neighborhood, church, and community can be the saving grace for a person taking care of someone with Alzheimer's or dementia. Even though she may not ask for help, she will need others to get through this time in her life. The important part is for someone to set up a schedule to spread out the help. When we all visit or help at once, we are actually adding more stress to the care provider. We, in a team effort, can make a huge difference.

How to Give a Helping Hand

- Do the caregiver's laundry.

- Schedule people to drop off food every other day.

- Mow the caregiver's lawn (don't offer, just do it).

- Ask if there is anything you can get for her when you go to the grocery store

- Take the person with dementia on a country drive or to a ball game, so the care provider can take a break.

- Offer to stay with the person with dementia so the care provider can run errands, get her hair done, visit a friend.

- Give the caregiver meals that can be put in the freezer and then easily cooked in the oven.

- Mail her movie tickets or restaurant certificates anonomously.

- Offer to pick up her kids from sports or afternoon activities.

- Clean the caregiver's house and do the dishes.

- Share your garden vegetables.

- Take care of her loved one so she can have a night off.

People usually have difficulty accepting help and will refuse initially, but keep persisting. The first six months after a person's loved one has been diagnosed is usually the time when she needs you the most. She is adjusting to this new understanding and needs time to make necessary changes. A good way to help with laundry or cleaning inside the house is to find out when she will be out of the house so she doesn't have to watch you help. It's too easy for her to feel guilty when we help while she is watching.

Whenever possible, help anonomously. When offering
help, reassure and say, "You are my friend. I care about you,
so please let me help."

When we truly care for ourselves, it becomes possible to care far
more profoundly about other people. The more alert and sensi-
tive we are to our own needs, the more loving and generous we
can be toward others.

—Eda LeShan

New-Found Way to Nurture Yourself
and Tasks Others Can Help You With

Conclusion

I would like to elaborate on the vision I talked about in the beginning of this book. When I became an activity director at a special care Alzheimer's unit, I didn't have any experience working in a nursing home and knew little about the disease. In other words, I didn't have a preconceived notion of how it should be; I just created what I thought the people needed. I believe this is why my ideas have been so effective. Once you have a clear vision and start focusing on that vision, the steps to get there will begin to evolve naturally. Fighting for something or someone else will give you the determination, faithfulness, and passion you need to succeed. It's not easy, and there are days when you'll want to quit. But you'll have your purpose, your vision to fall back on. Fight for your passion!

If you see a wall in front of you, find out what the materials are in the wall and figure out how to tear it down. Keep using your tools to dig into the wall. When you find a treasure that creates a moment of joy, it will create a hole in the wall for you to see through. Then you can get a glimpse at the new vision. Look beyond the wall (the disease) and focus on the person who needs you. Love and care with a genuine heart. That's when you will fly, feel warmth, and start smelling the daisies.

Every moment is a memory.
—Rosemary Brackey

I want to thank you, Lord,
for being close to me so far this day.

With your help I haven't been impatient, lost my temper,
been grumpy, judgmental, or envious of anyone.

BUT
I will be getting out of bed in a minute, and I think
I will really need your help then!
Amen

Bibliography

Freeman, Arthur. "Spirituality, Well-being, and Ministry." *JPC* 52, no. 1 (spring 1998): 7.

Johnson, Barbara. *Boomerang Joy: Joy That Goes Around, Comes Around.* Zondervan Publishing House, 1998.

Jones, Moyra. *Gentlecare: Changing the Experience of Alzheimer's Disease in a Positive Way.* Moyra Jones Resources, 1996.

Kitterman, Ron. "Spiritual Well-being and Alzheimer's Disease," 1998.

McKim, Donald K. *God Never Forgets: Faith, Hope, and Alzheimer's Disease.* Ed. Westminister John. Louisville, Ky.: Knox Press, 1997.

Nelson, Dawn. "Massaging Victims of Alzheimer's Disease: Communication and Caring through Touch." *Massage* 53 (Jan/Feb 1995): 24-29.

Pain Management was written by Lori Linton Nelson, RN, MN, PMHNP, Benedictine Institute for Long Term Care, Mt. Angel, Oregon. She is working on a grant through the Hartford Institute on Geriatric Nursing at New York University to improve pain management delivery in the elderly population.

The Power of Touch, Spread the Holidays throughout the Year, and Sexuality were written by Jeanne Yordi. She is the Program Coordinator for the Alzheimer's Association Mid-Iowa Chapter.

Index

Activities, 23, 31, 59, 75, 79, 91, 126, 131, 140, 146

Being in someone else's room, 30, 80

Development level, 4, 160, 169

Enhanced independence, 55, 68, 85, 88, 129, 161

Fragmented sleeping, 152

Getting robbed, 52

Hallucinations, 52

Helping hands, 174

Hitting, 151

How to get answers, 44, 47, 55

I want to go home, 17, 20, 27, 82, 143

Incontinence, 34, 98

Losing items, 79, 151

Loss of depth perception, 49

Loss of emotional control, 150

Memory loss, 3, 9, 13, 20, 33, 169

Pain, 156

Repeating, 3, 20, 31

Sexuality, 154

Triggering memories, 44, 48, 75, 79, 82, 85, 91, 147, 170

Wandering, 150

Wearing someone else's clothes, 30

When you don't understand them, 41

Meet the Author

After graduating from Iowa State University with a degree in interior design, my husband and I moved to Oregon to begin our lives together. I soon learned that interior design wasn't filling my inner desire to help others. I began focusing on what would make me happy and knew I enjoyed being around older people. Little did I realize they would give me treasures I will use for a lifetime. Being an activ-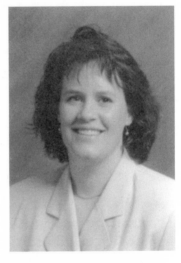ity director for a special care Alzheimer's unit helped me realize my natural gift to create positive outcomes. "

Progressing in my work, I set up three Alzheimer's facilities, attended many educational conferences, began presenting educational seminars, and established by business, Enhanced Moments. Enhanced Moments gives me the freedom to do what I love to do—make a difference by helping others. My underlining passion is to share my enthusiasm and knowledge with others so together, we can create many moments of joy.

Two years after I started my business my mom found a heart I made in Sunday School when I was seven years old. In the middle it said, *Love is . . .* I wrote, "Knowing Jesus,

Helping Mom and Dad, Helping make the bed, Helping old people."

God has planted this gift and prepared me for this journey. I encourage all people, young and old, to discover your "gift" and use it to make a difference in the lives of others.

Joys are our wings!

If you are interested in having Jolene Brackey speak to your organization or would like the educational videotape "Creating Moments of Joy," please contact:

Enhanced Moments
P.O. Box 383
Polk City, Iowa 50226
e-mail: moments@commongroup.net
www.enhancedmoments.com

I'd love to hear from readers who have had success creating special moments of joy, so that we could include them in future editions of this book. Your sharing will really help others to help their loved ones. Please contact me at the above address.